HEALTH EXPLORED

DR. MIKE WAHL PHD

WITH PHOTOGRAPHY BY BRAEDEN KING

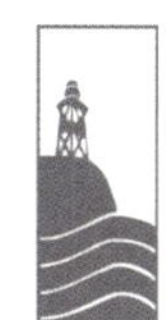

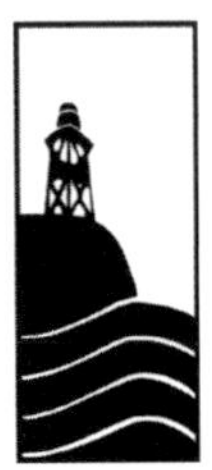

Breakwater Books
P.O. Box 2188, St. John's, NL, Canada, A1C 6E6
www.breakwaterbooks.com

A CIP catalogue record for this book is available from Library and Archives Canada.

ISBN 9781778530418 (hardcover)

Cover Photograph: *The author in front of volcanic Mount Taranaki, New Zealand*
Photographs: [page 3] *Mike Wahl at the Tiger's Nest Temple in Bhutan*; [page 5] *Lodhi Gardens, India*

Page Layout: Beth Oberholtzer, Oberholtzer Design Inc.

Printed and bound in Canada

We acknowledge the support of the Canada Council for the Arts.

We acknowledge the financial support of the Government of Canada through the Department of Heritage and the Government of Newfoundland and Labrador through the Department of Tourism, Culture, Arts, and Recreation for our publishing activities.

Breakwater Books is committed to choosing papers and materials for our books that help to protect our environment. To this end, this book is printed on a recycled paper and other sources that are certified by the Forest Stewardship Council®.

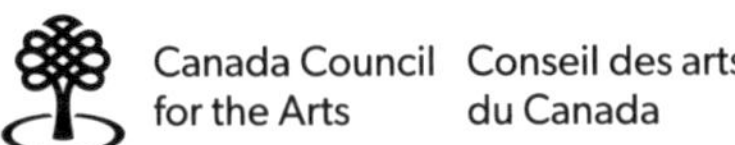

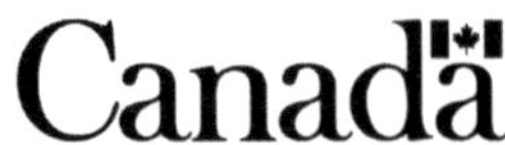

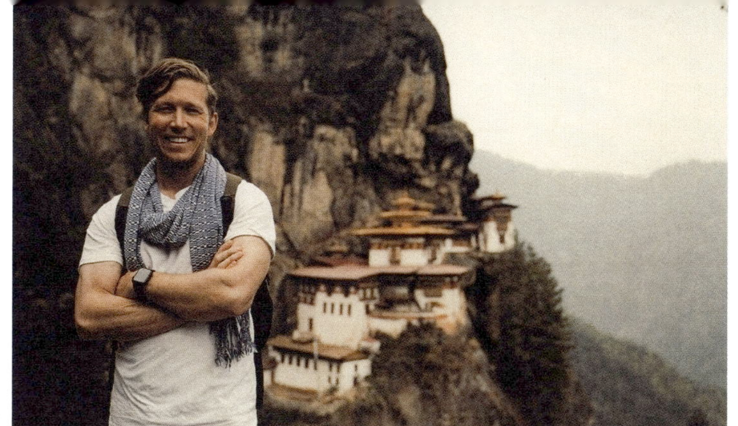

foreword

I have had the pleasure and honour to be a supervisor, colleague, and friend of Dr. Mike Wahl for over twenty years. Mike's life journey has brought him an appreciation of both the simplicity and complexity of life's struggles for happiness, healing, and humanity. This book carves a similar journey. Mike began his career focused on fitness and performance and training, but he soon realized that being fit does not always translate into happiness and contentment. As a lifelong teacher, Mike aims to share his personal journey, enriched by diverse global perspectives.

Mike takes us on a circuitous journey around the world, starting and ending in his own backyard of the province of Newfoundland and Labrador. From Newfoundland, the journey brings us first to a surf therapy program in New Zealand where we learn about the therapeutic essence of water that mimics the ebb and flow of our lives.

Travelling on to India and Bhutan, a typical Westerner would be surprised to discover the School of Happiness and a country that actually employs a statistical measure of Gross National Happiness. The contentment associated with the pursuit of selfless actions is not a primary or typical objective of the average Westerner but learning the law of cause and effect can bring greater balance and peace in our lives.

You would think that we all have an ikigai or "reason for being," but unlike the Okinawans, we often do not take time for this type of important contemplation. The pursuit of a purposeful life may be a major contributor to the great number of centenarians in this part of the world.

While in Tokyo, we are reminded of the need to not just be in nature but to experience and be with nature. Similar truths are to be found elsewhere around the world. In Costa Rica, you will meet centenarians who emphasize that longevity is not just about the length of our years but the depth of our connections. We need to have a Pura Vida, or pure life, philosophy rooted in work but nurtured by play.

When travelling through the Sahara Desert and Atlas Mountains of Morocco, we are told that the greatest lessons come from the simplest moments. In the West, we might say: "You need to slow down and smell the flowers." While in Morocco, you are warned, "If you are in a rush, then you are already dead."

As Mike takes us on this diverse journey, we discover common threads that unite different locations, cultures, and people. Our pursuit of optimal health and longevity, while important, should not overshadow our quest for happiness, wellness, and contentment. There is no one-size-fits-all approach to this journey. We are physical, mental, and spiritual beings, and all three aspects need to be harmoniously integrated in our lives. Mike will help you explore the different pathways that have been successful for others around the world to elevate all aspects of one's being and offer some insightful suggestions on how you can as well.

I know you will enjoy this journey!

— David G. Behm, PhD

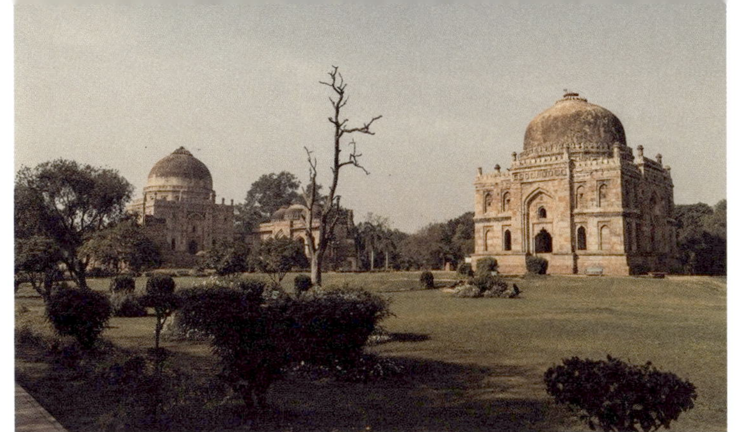

contents

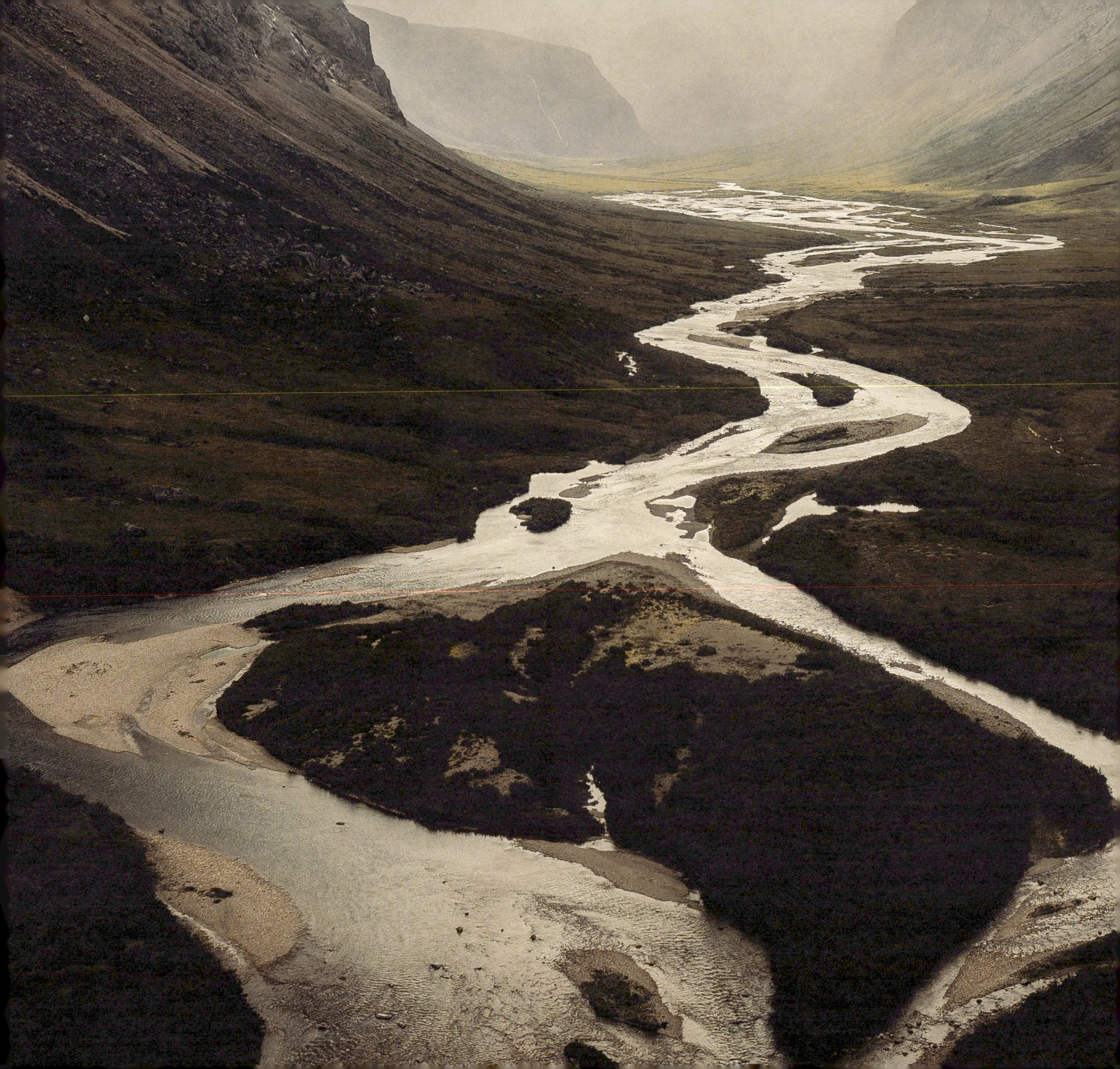

A BRAIDED RIVER

My mother always said that life is like a braided river that weaves a route toward its desired destination. My journey has been an exploration of health and humanity that has taken me around the world. This is my story, braided together with a collection of the lessons I've learned from those who have skillfully navigated the currents of a life well lived.

AWAKENING

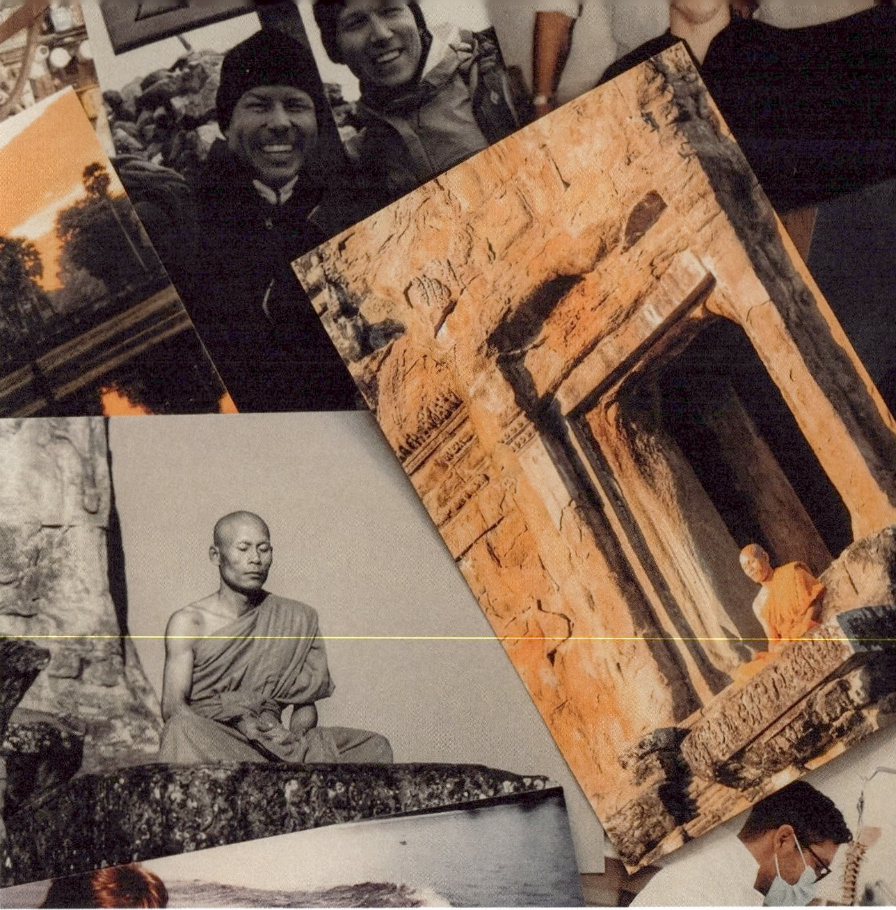

It's morning in this concrete jungle, and the monotone view dulls my senses. I stand in my corner office of a looming skyscraper in Toronto, overlooking the iconic CN Tower and the big city skyline dotted with similar skyscrapers, as a memory rises inside me. It was in Cambodia, where, one clear day, I watched the rising sun catch the sky on fire as it climbed over Angkor Wat. I was sitting with strangers on a stone staircase in the crimson light while a solitary monk meditated on a vine-covered perch high above us. As the sun warmed his face, his eyes never opened to break his practice, not even to glimpse at the majesty of the scene. I wondered what state of mind he had achieved to choose a colourless calm over striking beauty.

Breaking from memory, I turn to look at the desk in my office, where pamphlets on mindfulness apps for smart phones and self-care checklists are scattered, and I shake my head. This isn't the life I envisioned; my heart yearns for genuine connections and alignment with what I believe, something that my career in wellness had once offered but has slipped away unwittingly over time.

It's not the first time I've felt disconnected from what I believe and what I'm selling. In my corporate role, I have often recommended solutions like office stretches, knowing they are merely superficial fixes for a lifestyle detached from our true nature. I have learned this during my own travel and life experiences, such as on a several-week trek to Machu Picchu I made in memory of my father. Accompanied by my cousin David, I journeyed through the heart of the mountains, witnessing traditional methods of healing and local customs. We were awe-struck by the Andean snow-capped peaks and the star-filled night skies. We made an offering to Mother Earth during a Pachamama ceremony on the shores of a glacier lake and watched the smoke from the ritual spiral into the blue sky above. Each step on the path was a step toward introspection and connection with the past, honouring a family legacy of adventure. These moments were transformative, transcending the usual metrics of calories and heart rates, and were not bound by the prescription of conventional wellness.

My high-rise Toronto office, a symbol of the corporate success I had always strived for, feels oddly hollow. And this introspective morning marks the beginning of a new chapter in my life, steering me back to my roots of curiosity and exploration.

My corporate workweek in the big city is over, and I head back to Newfoundland. When the doors of the airport slide open, I smell the salty air of the island I call home. There is nothing like the feeling of coming home. Back in the comforting embrace of my community, amidst conversations and laughter, a friend casually asks what I want to do next. I don't have an easy answer, but his question lingers in my mind.

[previous page] A braided river in the Torngat Mountains of Northern Labrador
[above] The colourless calm of a monk during sunrise—detail from one of the author's memory collages

BEGINNINGS

My journey in health started with an analog childhood of tree forts and skateboarding. My mother, a physical education teacher, collegiate diver, and provincial gymnastics coach, greatly influenced my early years. My father, a geologist, would set up mining camps in the Canadian North or call us "collect" from pay phones in some country we would have to look up on a map. As kids, my sister and I enjoyed homemade snacks like "beetles on a log," a creative camouflaging of healthy food—our celery sticks buried in peanut butter and topped with insect-mimicking raisins. It didn't stop there; we would have push-up competitions in the living room and ski and bike together as a family. I was lucky to have that influence at home during my formative years. Little did my mother know, I would follow in her footsteps as an educator and an entrepreneur.

I excelled academically and played sports, but my parents never pushed me into competition, allowing me to find my own way. I was a late bloomer, and in my early teens, while my friends grew taller, I remained the shortest in my class, driving me to prove my athletic worth.

I remember rushing down the long junior high hallway toward the gymnasium, where the coaches posted the final cuts for the basketball and volleyball teams. I arrived with my troop of friends and stared at the lists of newly named players. Scrolling through the alphabetical order to W, my name was absent, and the disappointment crushed me. My friends had made both teams, and I had made neither. I held back tears as I felt the heartache of failure for the first time.

But my parents, understanding the challenges of my late development, encouraged me to stay involved but in a different role—as a team manager. Initially, I perceived the role as reserved for "geeks," but my parents helped me see its opportunities. I could practise with the team if someone was absent, learn the plays, and get to know the coaches and players. I embraced the role, taking stats, assisting with drills, and becoming a junior coach. My perseverance paid off the following year when my name made both team lists, with the coaches appointing me captain for both squads. Of all my most formative experiences, this one taught me the value of hard work and dedication at a young age.

I must have been a stubborn kid, as adversity seemed only to fuel my early progress. Our teams had weight training sessions as part of our dryland training; I was invariably the underdog. Despite being smaller than the rest of my teammates, I never let that deter me, even when common sense would encourage me to take a step back. As is often the case, the boys organized a bench-press contest. Joel—almost six feet tall in Grade 8 with a scruffy mustache—was the clear favourite to win.

The contest started with just the bar, then the weight was gradually increased. Weighing only ninety-five pounds myself, I struggled to lift sixty pounds and was then faced with an eighty-pound target. But I was determined to try. As I positioned my hands on the bar, ready for the lift, my best friend, Daran, who was spotting me, counted to three and I lifted the bar off. Daran steadied it, asking, "You good . . .?" as he watched my arms sway under the weight. In response, I grunted, "Nah," intending to say no, but it sounded too much like an affirmative "yeah." Misinterpreting my response, Daran let go, and suddenly, my arms faltered under the weight. The bar started descending toward my head. In a desperate effort, I managed to slow its fall, narrowly

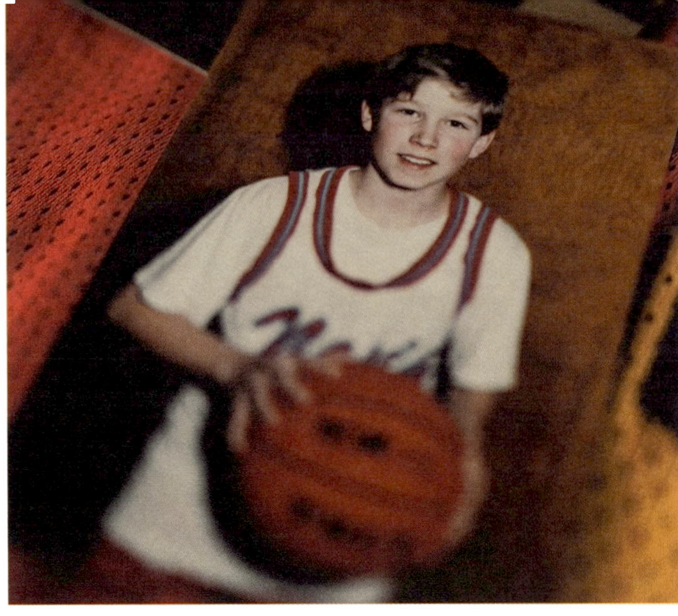

avoiding serious injury. The other boys quickly intervened, lifting the bar off me. At that moment, I could almost hear them coining the nickname "80" in their minds.

In certain circles, I'm still known as "80" to this day, and though I initially despised it, it ignited my passion for weightlifting. Returning home with the mark of the bar on my forehead, I recounted the episode to my parents, expressing my desire to get stronger and get some weights for home. My father had faced similar challenges as a skinny kid and deeply empathized with my situation. My mother, the former physical education teacher, was happy to support any healthy activity. The next day, we started transforming our basement into a gym. My father installed twelve-by-twelve mirrors across the back wall to create a reflective surface for monitoring my form. Soon after, a home gym set-up arrived with free weights and bars. It was the most heartfelt support I could have asked for, and I was lucky to grow up in a family that provided such encouragement.

I worked out daily with meticulous routines, complete with spreadsheets of reps and weights, recorded fitness shows, and pored over Arnold Schwarzenegger's *Encyclopedia of Modern Bodybuilding*. This regimen became my identity, boosting my confidence immensely. By Grade 10, I designed workout plans for my friends, including the titan, Joel.

Fast forward to my first university job, in which I was a shoe tag checker in the University of New Brunswick weight room—a job I had secured based on my affinity for working out. My main task was to ensure that each gym member displayed their hefty blue shoe tag—a seemingly trivial but necessary gym policy. Day after day, I was stationed in a chair by the door, a post that quickly proved dull and monotonous, especially for someone with my energetic nature.

However, this job had its silver linings. The idle hours spent in that chair sparked a new direction in my fitness journey. I began interacting more with the gym members, offering tips and guidance. Before I knew it, I was informally training people, sharing the knowledge and techniques I had honed over the years in my basement and now in the classroom as a kinesiology student.

By the time I turned nineteen, I had snagged the enviable gig of being a beer rep, a job that came with the golden ticket of free drinks. This role swiftly taught me about the community dynamics of the university: I learned that free beer is a magnet for various social circles, particularly for the varsity athletes on the men's hockey team. When it occurred to the team that I could also get free beer on other campuses where they travelled for games, a strategy huddle broke out in the bar, culminating in a proposal for me to join their support staff. In the competitive world of my kinesiology peers, landing the role of hockey team trainer was a coveted achievement. Remarkably, I clinched this position, perhaps not as much by merit but by leveraging my unique influence on the team's bar expenditures.

My career seemed to be one convenient coincidence after another. The work with the hockey team landed me a role with a world-famous hockey strength coach on the outskirts of New York City. After two years of hard work, I earned the opportunity to move back to Canada to complete a master's in kinesiology at Memorial University, a decision made easier by a day I will never forget.

On the morning of September 11, 2001, standing in that gym north of New York City, the world around us changed irreversibly. I recall receiving an email confirming admission to Memorial University from Dr. David Behm at around 8:30 a.m. that day. Excitedly, I shared this news with my client during our training session that morning when, suddenly, the televisions all switched to the news; we looked up to see the World Trade Center on fire following the first plane's impact. We watched in disbelief as the second tower was struck before our eyes, and that was when panic set in. We were only a few kilometres from the city, and many of our professional clients worked in the Twin Towers. In the ensuing tragedy, we learned that one gym member had lost her husband in the attack, while two others mourned the loss of family members. The morning after the attack, riding my motorcycle along I-95 was surreal—the usually bustling highway was eerily deserted with the city's bridges closed. Meanwhile, the opposite lane was a stream of ambulances and military vehicles rushing north to Connecticut hospitals. That moment crystallized my decision to come home to Canada.

A few months later, I was settled into Newfoundland and eager to make my mark; I distributed meticulously crafted workout plans to the coaches of every one of Memorial University's sports teams and offered gym sessions for any athletes looking for help.

The university appointed me the varsity kinesiologist, entrusting me with a dingy corner of the equipment room, jammed between the floor hockey sticks and soccer balls. The clinic had a half-broken massage table next to a makeshift garbage container I outfitted with a water-draining valve. I remember wheeling the Frankenstein garbage bin to the gym doors and shovelling it full of snow at the start of each day. Hours later, preferably melted, it would serve as a creative ice bath for the varsity athletes in our improvised clinic.

This role eventually expanded beyond athletes as local business people sought my expertise. Since these consultations had to occur outside the walls of the university, I began looking for a location to work.

I teamed up with an athlete and entrepreneur to create Definitions, a unique boutique gym in historic downtown St. John's. Our concept, blending personal training with a focus on health, was initially met with skepticism, particularly from bankers who found our membership and pricing model unconventional.

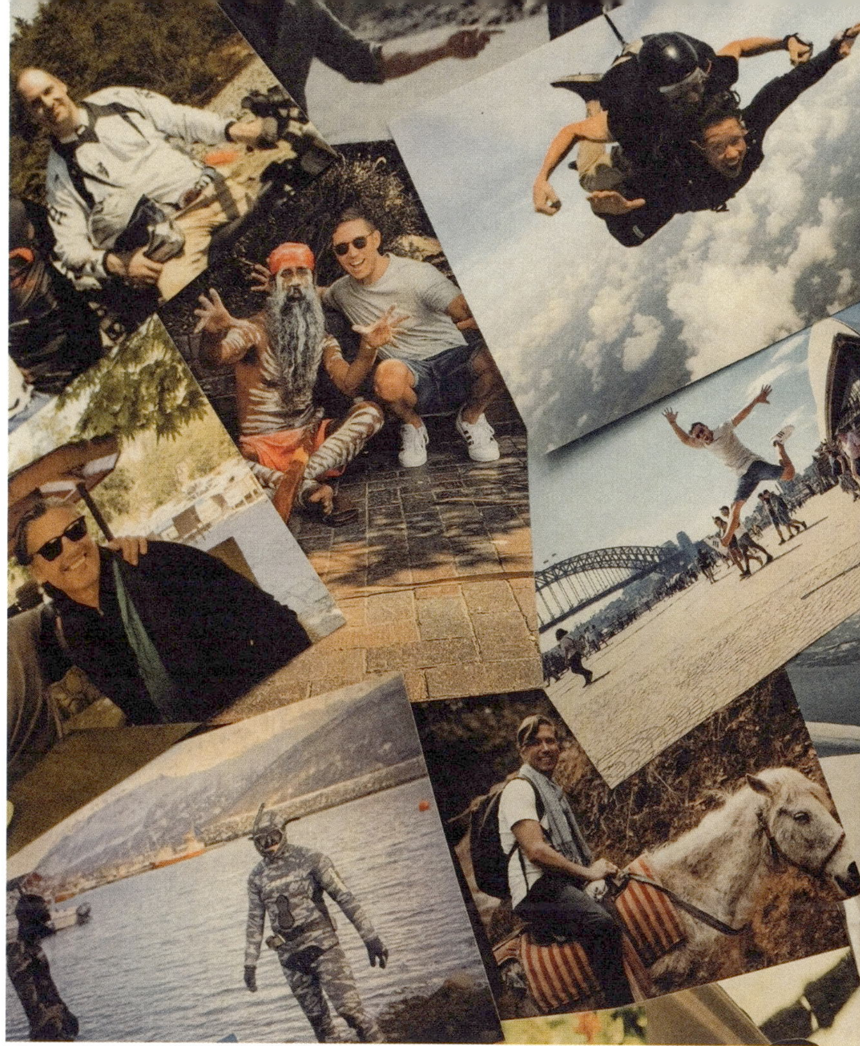

Financial challenges were significant in the early stages. Personal sacrifices, like selling my car and moving into my business partner's basement, which boasted a six-foot ceiling, were part of the reality of entrepreneurship. I remember the excitement when I could afford to upgrade my sleeping arrangements from an air mattress to a futon.

Without athletes to rehab, I started helping captains of industry instead of hockey teams. One such client asked me to visit his workplace to help with his employees' injuries. These employees, later coined "industrial athletes," called oil rigs, mining sites, shipyards, and factories their homes. Another door had opened in my life, but this one was different.

[opposite] Practice makes good enough—a Junior Varsity accomplishment
[above] From sea to sky—a collection of memories from far off places

HARSH ENVIRONMENTS

I'll never forget the sound of the loud clink as the latch opens on a solid metal marine door. I'm dressed in a bright orange survival suit that I donned right after we finished the pre-flight stretching program my company had designed. We put our earplugs in and stand in line. It is always a crap shoot to pinch and roll them just enough to slide them into your ears before they expand again quickly. I hear the whooshing sound of my heartbeat in my ears; my blood pressure spikes as I stand in uncomfortable silence with ten other men, hoping to be able to get home. The door swings open, and the new crew enters; handshakes and muffled conversations occur before the helideck operator motions us to head out the door. We clamber up the yellow metal stairs, and before I know it, I am staring across a helideck over 100 metres above the angry Atlantic Ocean.

I pass my duffle bag to the first man in the line of ten, all clad in high-visibility red coveralls; my other hand clings to the frozen metal handrail. The helicopter's blades whir noisily in front of me as fuel hoses are unlatched and fire teams stand on the ready.

My bag moves down the chain of men, each bracing themselves against the biting wind, until it finally reaches the helicopter and is tossed in with the other passengers' luggage. I survey the churning waves below, their whitecaps stark against the cold February sea. Exhaustion weighs on me; my seven-day visit had been a marathon of little sleep and constant activity as I tried to work with each member of a crew that works round-the-clock shifts. I'd made numerous friends, and by the time of my departure, many were seeking advice about their health. It was a rewarding yet challenging dynamic to navigate.

My gaze is fixed on the amber light on the deck, knowing it could turn red at any second, cancelling our flight and stranding me on this oil rig in the North Atlantic for another week. Just within the weather limits, this flight is my long-awaited ticket home.

"Let's go, buddy," the first man in the chain urged, breaking me free of my thoughts. I move along the human lifeline, each person offering a hand or an arm to steady me against the gusting wind. Each crew member says their goodbyes. "See ya next time, Mikey," and "Be good pal," and then the ultimate salute: a head twist nod, that only a Newfoundlander could understand. I make my way to the helicopter, each step cautious on the wind-battered helideck as I walk on the

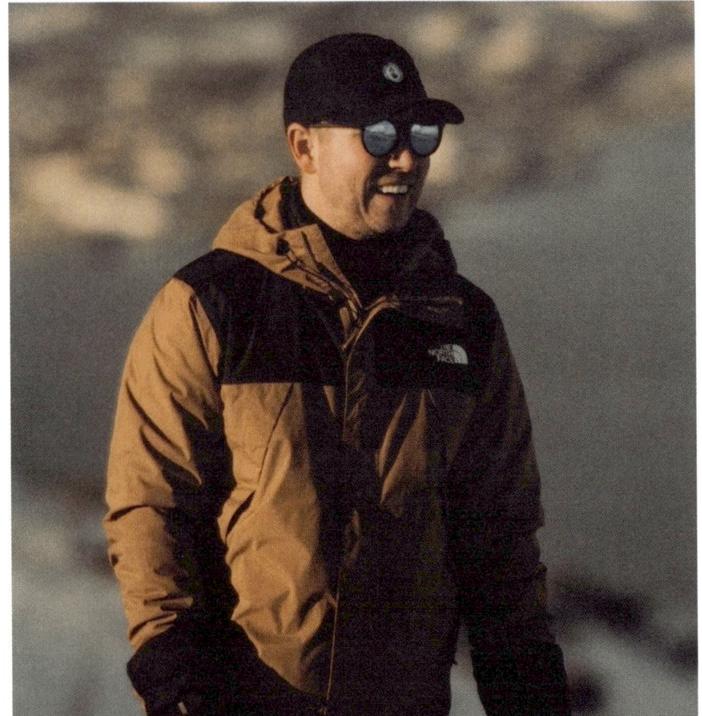

netting provided underfoot for traction. Climbing aboard, I strap into my seat, donning my extra ear protection and zipping the seals on my flight suit. The flight crew's arrival in the helicopter signals the final check—a thumbs-up and a seat belt confirmation.

As the door closes, the howling wind is silenced, and my eyes flicker back to the light on the flight deck. The helicopter's blades accelerate, the aircraft shudders, and we are airborne. The light switches to red as soon as we leave the surface, a sign that this is the last flight for the next few days. A collective sigh of relief sweeps through the cabin; we are eager to be reunited with our families after a long absence.

During this portion of my career, I spent over 400 days on oil rigs all around the world. Our company set up offices in Aberdeen, Scotland, and Houston, Texas, and with our niche secured, the business expanded rapidly.

It was during this time that personal challenges emerged. Loss, turmoil, and struggles marked a period of profound change in my home and business lives. Mental health became a focus of my routine, and I learned to appreciate the challenges many people face daily. Up to that point in life, my road had been one with few obstacles, so although uncomfortable and foreign, the experience was formative.

My idea of health as being merely physical had faded, replaced instead with an appreciation that health is a much more complex puzzle.

I surrounded myself with good people in my business, committing to the philosophy that you are the average of the five people you spend the most time with. Mentors emerged like Dr. Hassan Khalili, psychologist and author of *A Life Spent Listening*, who rehabilitated my mind and soul, and Stephen Henley, an oil and gas leader and client turned best friend, who provided guidance and support in both personal and professional aspects.

A few years later, I received a notification on my phone while I was walking downtown in St. John's. It was a LinkedIn message. Reading it, I stopped in my tracks, quickly checking the source to ensure it was legitimate. The message was an invitation to join a group of business investors for breakfast to discuss the acquisition of my company. Shortly after that meeting, our company was purchased, and I found myself overlooking the Toronto skyline from that corner office.

I was caught in a whirlwind of travel, clocking in over seventy flights per year, and I faced many challenges integrating our unique services into the new company's more significant, ever-evolving structure. After another more extensive merger, the issues only compounded as the new parent company transformed our boutique business into part of a vast, impersonal corporate entity.

I soon discovered that within the corporate realm, decisions were often driven more by the health of the stock price rather than that of the clients. This realization hit me hard the day the new head of the company visited our St. John's location, which still proudly bore a sign with the name Definitions—a testament to our roots as one of the last remaining independently operated businesses in the wider group. His visit, marked by an attempt to charm our staff with small stuffed animals and keychains, took a sobering turn when he casually mentioned removing the "Dimensions" sign from our door. In that moment, I witnessed the culture I had meticulously built over nearly two decades begin to crumble. It was a poignant reminder of the vast difference between the values of a close-knit, independent business and a large, profit-driven corporation.

Shortly after, I exited the company, which meant saying goodbye to a job and an identity I had nurtured and grown for almost eighteen years. Leaving was a massive personal transition, a time for introspection and exploration as I focused less on work and more on areas of my life that were lacking. I began nurturing relationships, fostering hobbies, and prioritizing my health and recreation. This phase also ignited my desire to embark on projects that resonated more deeply with me and made a real difference.

[opposite] Overlooking winter

THE UNKNOWN

Though it was a period filled with uncertainty and fear, there was also a sense of excitement and liberation in charting a new course. I realized that I genuinely sought a life filled with meaningful connections and experiences, a stark contrast to the corporate lifestyle I had left behind. In some ways, this change was reassuring, a sign of maturing and personal growth and a means of wiping the slate clean.

I decided to travel again. These trips rekindled a deep-seated passion for exploration, but experiencing a place authentically was entirely new. Previously, my travel experiences had been confined mainly to structured environments—attending conferences, fulfilling work commitments, or ticking off tourist sites. This time, I needed it to be different. I wanted not just to visit places but to immerse myself in them, venturing off the beaten path and genuinely engaging with different cultures and lifestyles. I was learning to play again and live without the constant pressure of big business breathing down my neck.

In Australia, I toured the Gold Coast in a rented camper van, explored small towns, and took in the beautiful forests without a deadline. When I helped a friend build his new restaurant south of Brisbane and learned to shape surfboards with a Noosa legend, I was not just a visitor but a participant in the local community. Scuba diving in the Great Barrier Reef and seeing the devastation of bleaching reefs or encountering a pack of dingoes at Crescent Head wasn't just about ticking items off on a must-see checklist but connecting with nature in its rawest form.

One of my fondest memories of that trip is driving down an unknown route in the Blue Mountains using a hand-drawn map to find a non-descript driveway, then slowly climbing up it. A cabin and a guest house were supposed to be at the end of this dirt road. The Canadian family who lived there had heard I was passing through the area and invited me to stay for the night.

Arriving at the top of the driveway, the family warmly greeted me on their patio. Over a home-cooked dinner and a few bottles of wine, we talked about Canada. During our conversation, I felt an unexpected yearning for home. Despite being in a paradisiacal setting on the other side of the world, the familiar stories and laughter about our shared home stirred a deep longing within me.

The night extended into the early hours until I retired to the guest house built on the mountain's edge. The following morning, I awoke to a cabin bathed in golden sunlight. The valley below was veiled in mist, and blue-leaved eucalyptus trees sparkled with morning dew under the rising sun.

En route across the Pacific, I skateboarded down Waikiki Beach in Hawaii, thinking back to the surf shirts I would beg my parents for as a teenage skateboarder. I surfed Sunset Beach with an old friend and cruised the north shore in his 1960s VW Westfalia. During these moments, I felt a new tranquility from my experiences, derived from a recipe of simplicity and authenticity.

In Vietnam, travelling solo and making lifelong friends, I learned the value of unscripted adventures. I celebrated the Chinese New Year on an overnight train from Hanoi to Hue, toasting locals with an unknown liquor. I ate scorpions in Thailand and was foolishly over-confident in handling spicy food when I later ordered a meal with the "local" spice level, then spent the night curled in a ball in my hotel. I meandered through the redwood forests of British Columbia. I paddled through kelp beds to secret waves on my surfboard. I bagged my first Munro in

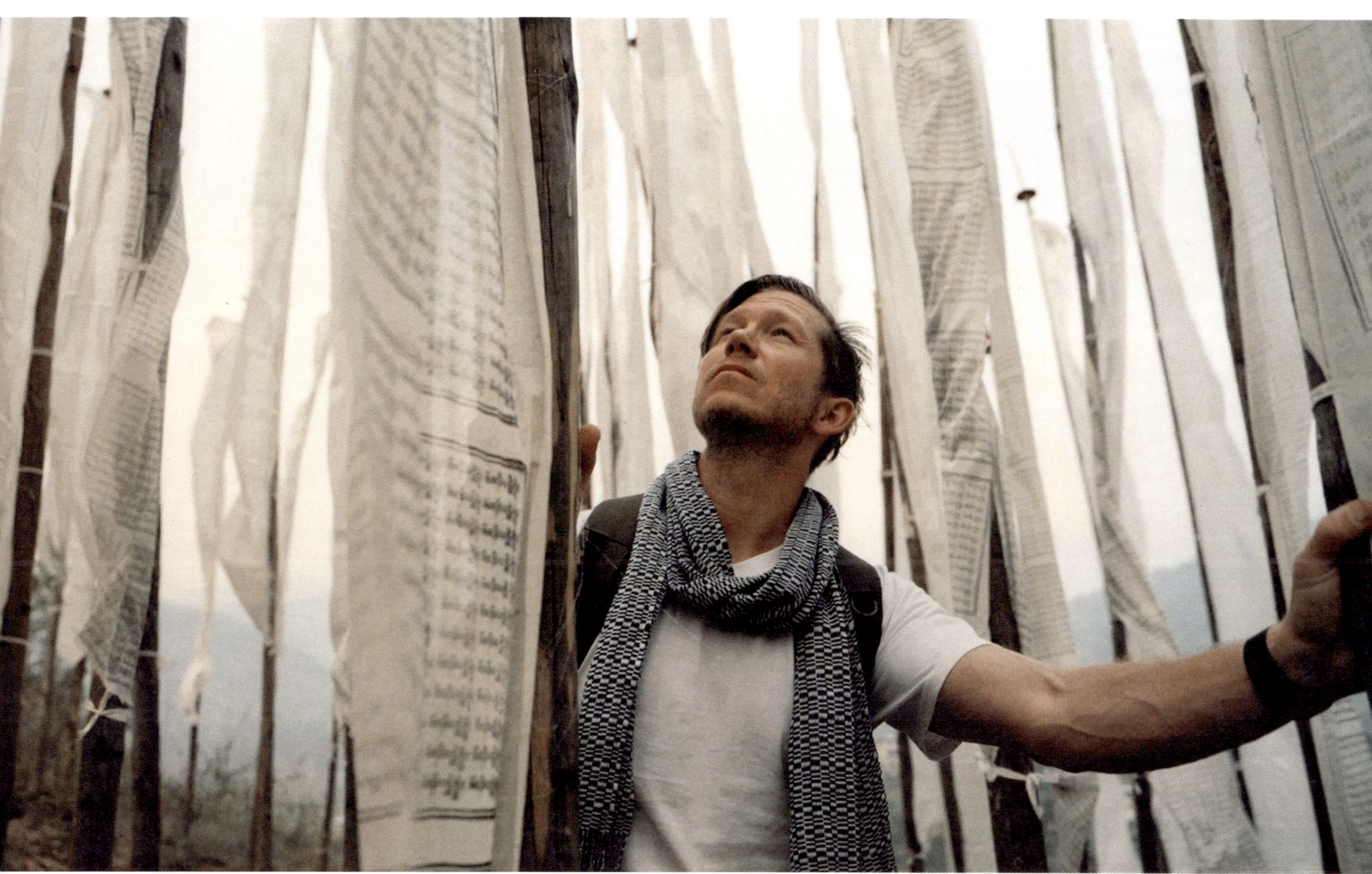

Scotland—a term given when you climb one of the mountains in the highlands my ancestors called home. But the day I learned the world was small was when I took the same picture as my university screensaver one sunny day in Greece.

These authentic adventures taught me the vast difference between seeing and truly experiencing a place. They resonated deeply with my personal growth and changed my perspective on what it means to explore and understand the world honestly. For me, the essence of travel lies in the unplanned moments, the personal stories, and the genuine interactions. After my travels, I found myself spiritually and intellectually renewed, inspired in ways I had never anticipated. And I found myself wanting more.

[above] A place of memory—wandering through prayer flags in Bhutan

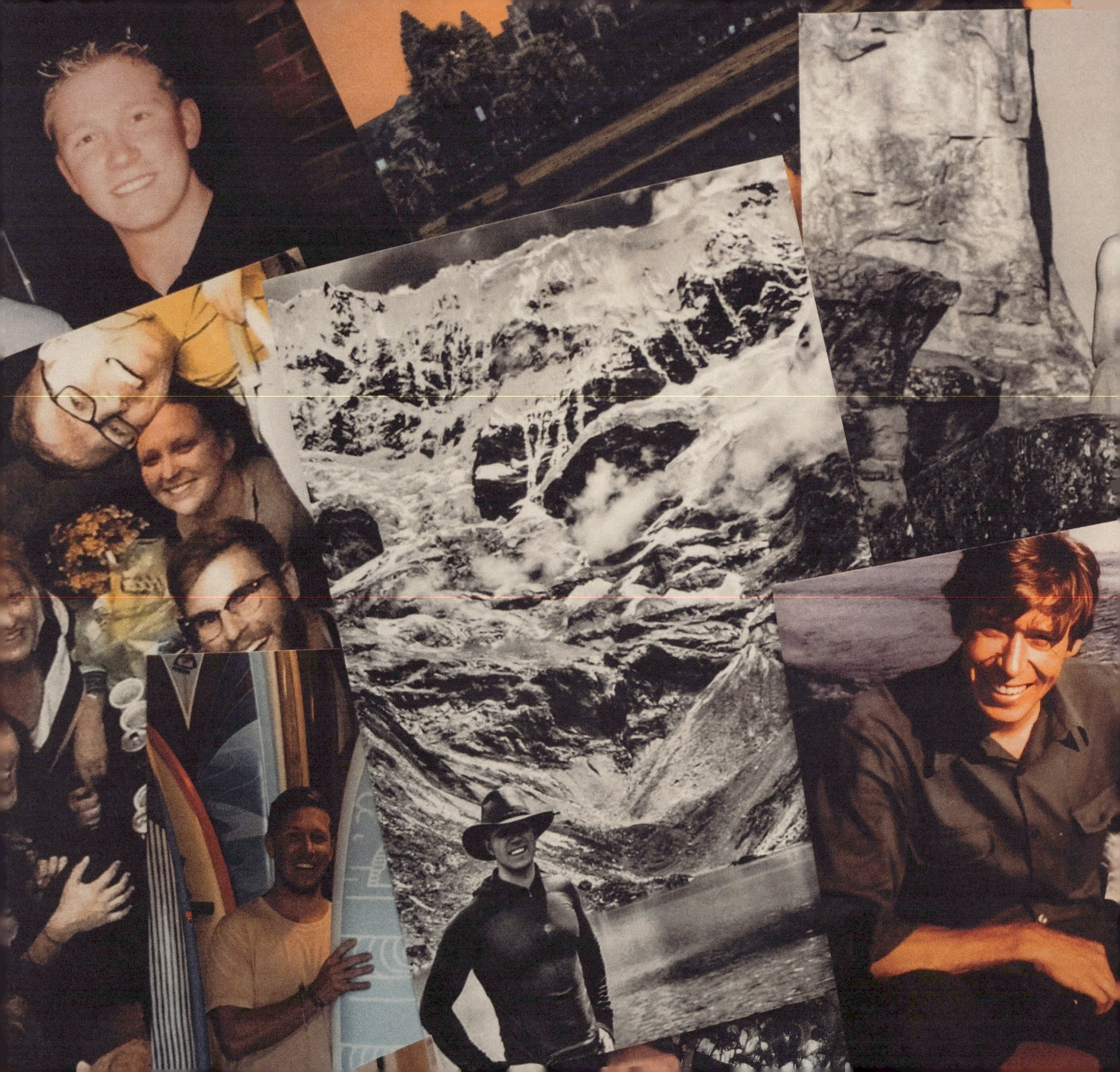

CLARITY, BALANCE, AND PURPOSE

Freed from corporate shackles, I embraced the opportunity to share my wellness philosophy with my community. This philosophy—rooted in a holistic view of health—goes beyond mere illness prevention. It challenges mainstream health trends of restrictive, often misleading narratives, instead advocating for a personalized, multifaceted approach to well-being.

This clarity led me to host a local radio show, an endeavour that quickly grew into more than just a platform for sharing knowledge. It became a calling, a means to connect with a broader audience and learn from experts in various health fields. The show's growth opened doors to new opportunities, including an unexpected offer to teach at Memorial University's medical school. Education, it turns out, has always been my true calling. From coaching in my youth to guiding others through my business, Definitions, I have always been a teacher. Counselling people on rigs, hosting a health-focused media program, and now working as a professor educating the next generation of physicians—all of this has been a fulfilling convergence of my academic pursuits and my career experience.

It also led to an opportunity to host a television show, *Health Explored*. Originally focused only on Newfoundland and Labrador, the show has grown in popularity and scope—which has, quite literally, opened the world to me. Alongside an amazing film crew, I've been able to travel to fascinating far-flung places all over the globe to explore how health and happiness, community and climate intersect. The show is an outgrowth of my passion to explore, expand my knowledge, and impart what I've learned about a complex health landscape to help people make informed individual decisions.

[opposite] Mountains, overnight trains and a dad to look up to
[right] Morning hike of Mount Manganui in New Zealand

This book is another way I want to share what I've come to know about health and happiness. This is an account of my personal journey, enriched by diverse global perspectives. In the following pages, you'll meet some of the amazing people who have shared their knowledge, wisdom, and ways of navigating the world with me. They are our guides on this journey.

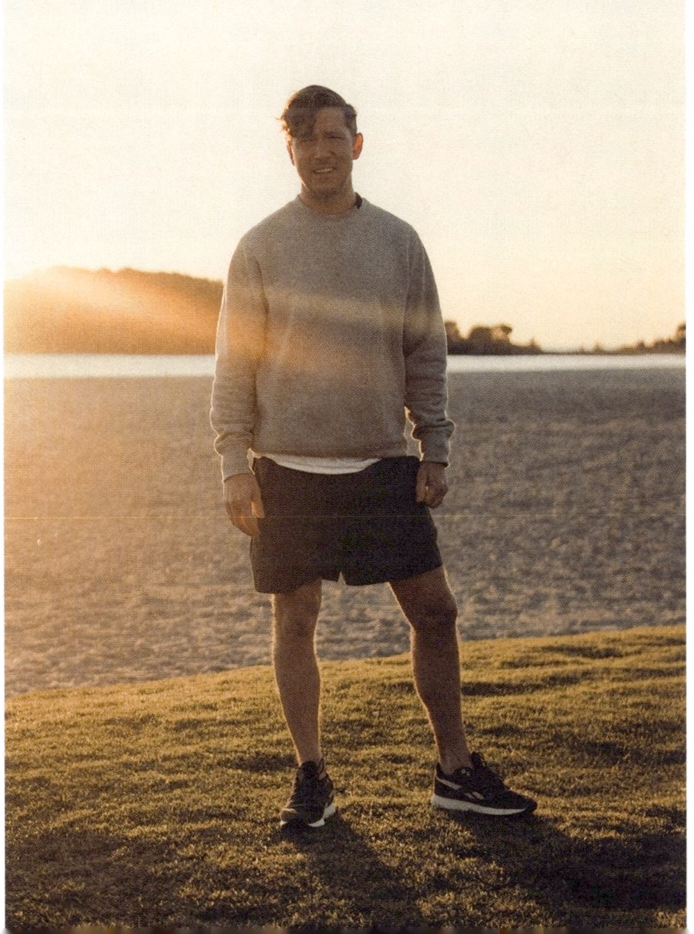

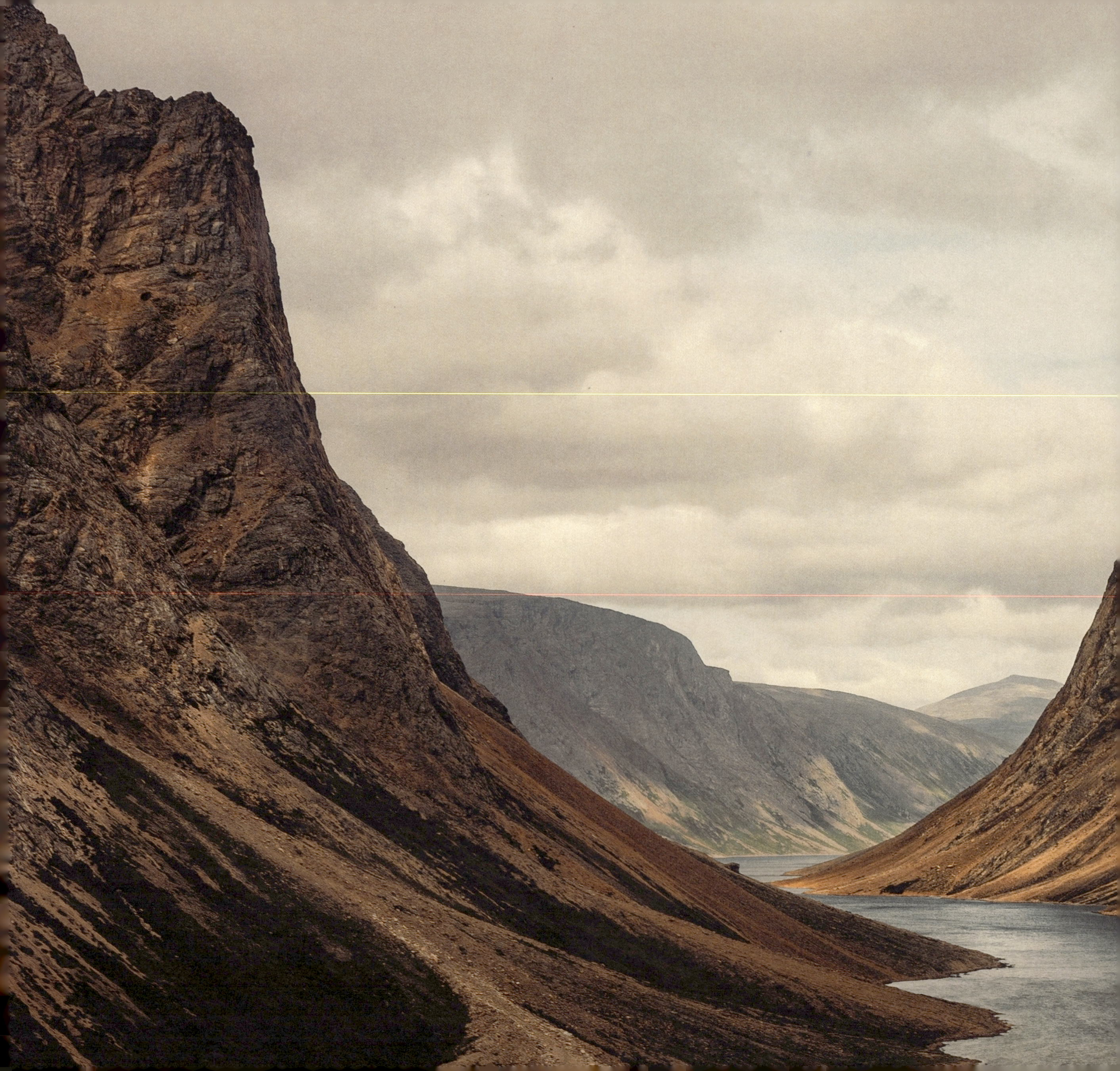

THE PLACE OF SPIRITS

The towering mountains in Torngat Mountains National Park hold a secret worth discovering. It's a nearly inaccessible location that whispers tales of the past and guidance for the future. Here, in the place the spirits call home, I reconnect with nature and learn the health secrets of this dramatic landscape.

LURING ME IN

On a dock that extends from the shoreline, my eyes fix on the bobber at the end of my line. Suddenly, it snaps downwards. It's on. The rod bends under the weight of an Arctic char, its power pulling the line away from me. I let the line run, feeling a sense of connection to the wild waters of Northern Labrador.

The char, a flash of silver in the darkening waters, makes a swift turn, heading back toward the dock. I reel in frantically, trying to keep the tension on the line as I haul the rod back over my shoulder, my eyes searching for any sign of my adversary. But the sun's reflection off the choppy water disguises the fish, turning the surface into a textured canvas of shimmering light.

Around me, the Torngat Mountains rise like ancient guardians, their peaks touching the sky. The cool, onshore breeze is fresh and untouched. I am in the home of Inuit legends, and I feel the untamed spirit of the land. Here, in this remote outpost, where nature remains pristine, I witness life thriving during the narrow window of summer.

It took less than a minute out here to hook the large char with a borrowed rod from Donovan, a teenage Inuk student and fisherman. Donovan has come north to immerse himself in the traditions of his ancestors and now stands beside me, offering guidance and coaching as I play my catch.

The cheers of my newfound northern friends ring out as I reel in the fish. In this moment, a permanent picture is taken in my mind that I'll revisit many times. I am immersed in what the Inuit call the place of spirits, and I feel mine awaken with the excitement of the catch and the beauty of the wilderness.

Few venture into the Torngat Mountains. At this moment, I'm glad it's just us out here. I hold up the char, which glistens in the remaining light of the day, and I know this experience is more than I had initially expected—it's a journey into a disappearing world and the most untouched of wonders.

On a planet that seems to be moving faster and faster, time in this place stands still. Getting lost in nature might be the key to finding balance and reconnecting with the natural world that eludes many of us.

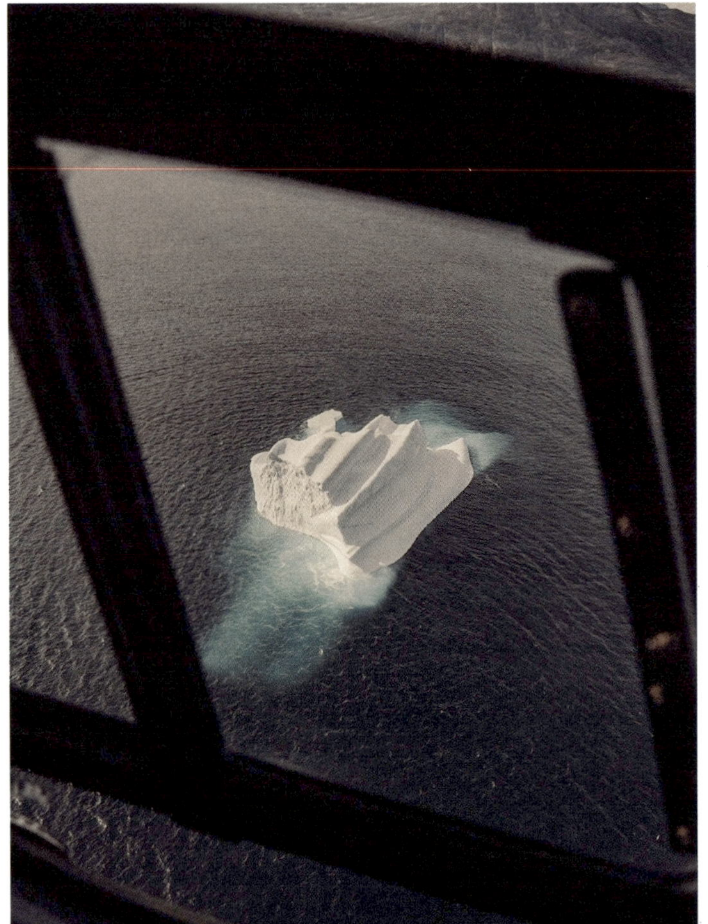

[previous page] Carved by Nature
[right] Icebergs from helicopters—entering the park

JOURNEY TO THE PLACE OF SPIRITS

How and why I am here stems from some advice from my mentor and friend, Dr. Hassan Khalili, author of *A Life Spent Listening*. Besides being a respected psychologist, "Doc" is also a world-class explorer. He has hiked across the Silk Road and Camino de Santiago, trekked through the Andes to Machu Picchu, summited Mount Kilimanjaro, and chased penguins in Antarctica. He sees nature as medicine for our minds and the abundance of it in our province and country as an untapped resource for health. As an adventurer and avid outdoorsman, he challenged me to expand my horizons and go further. He has encouraged me to immerse myself in nature and to see something that will change me forever. The Torngats fit that prescription perfectly.

The trip, organized in partnership with Provincial Airlines and Air Borealis, consists of me and the creative film crew of *Health Explored*: Braeden King, James MacKinnon and Liam Dawe.

At this point, we haven't travelled around the world—we haven't even left the province of Newfoundland and Labrador—yet it feels like we've been dropped into another world entirely. This province has more than a double-barrelled name; it has a dual personality. While most of the residents of Canada's easternmost province live, like I do, on the island of Newfoundland in the North Atlantic, about 27,000 people live in this vast place called Labrador on the mainland. Labrador has been home to Inuit and Innu people since time immemorial.

After a long few days of travel, we arrive on the abandoned airstrip at Saglek Bay, a narrow concrete patch in an otherwise untouched landscape. We unload our gear, talking with our fellow travellers for the first time as the prop engines slow. There's an Inuk craftsperson, a reporter and podcast host, some youth, and others coming to the park to reconnect with their culture. It's a small and privileged few who come to visit in the summer, and we are lucky enough to be among them.

As we stand outside in the cool air, the plane heads to the end of the runway, revealing a man in bright orange coveralls with a rifle slung over his shoulder. It now occurs to me that this man, who's a bear guard, will be one of our new best friends as reality, remoteness, and the vulnerability of our surroundings hit home. We are in a large valley with a small plateau that houses the runway and abandoned military buildings, which I learn are a favourite stomping ground for polar bears. The valley extends to the ocean, and in the distance, I see icebergs in the water. The sun reflects off the rocks, glistening with dew as the last of the morning fog burns away.

From the horizon, I hear a steady pulse of helicopter blades that take me out of the moment into the realization that we haven't even entered the park. I am already awestruck, and as the helicopter approaches, the pilot expertly spins it toward us as it seemingly floats to the ground. We are briefed on helicopter safety and load our gear into the metal bins attached to the landing bars. I clamber into the helicopter and don my headset. The propellers hum as the pilot prepares for takeoff, and before we know it, we are rising, angling forward and hurtling toward base camp. The wind makes the helicopter sway from side to side as it increases speed, and the ground flies by below in a blur.

We approach a mountain ridge, climb its face, and move over its summit like we're riding a roller coaster. Cresting the summit reveals a massive iceberg in the waters below. Everywhere I look, I see something breathtaking. We veer to the left down a bay, getting our first sight of the destination ahead: a small base camp of tents that reminds me of a moon colony or a secret outpost. My heart beats faster, and my face hurts from smiling. Taps on shoulders are generously supplied, and chatter fills the headsets as we all state the obvious. It's a struggle to communicate my excitement, resorting to unrestrained thumbs-ups and head-exploding hand gestures.

I'm in it now.

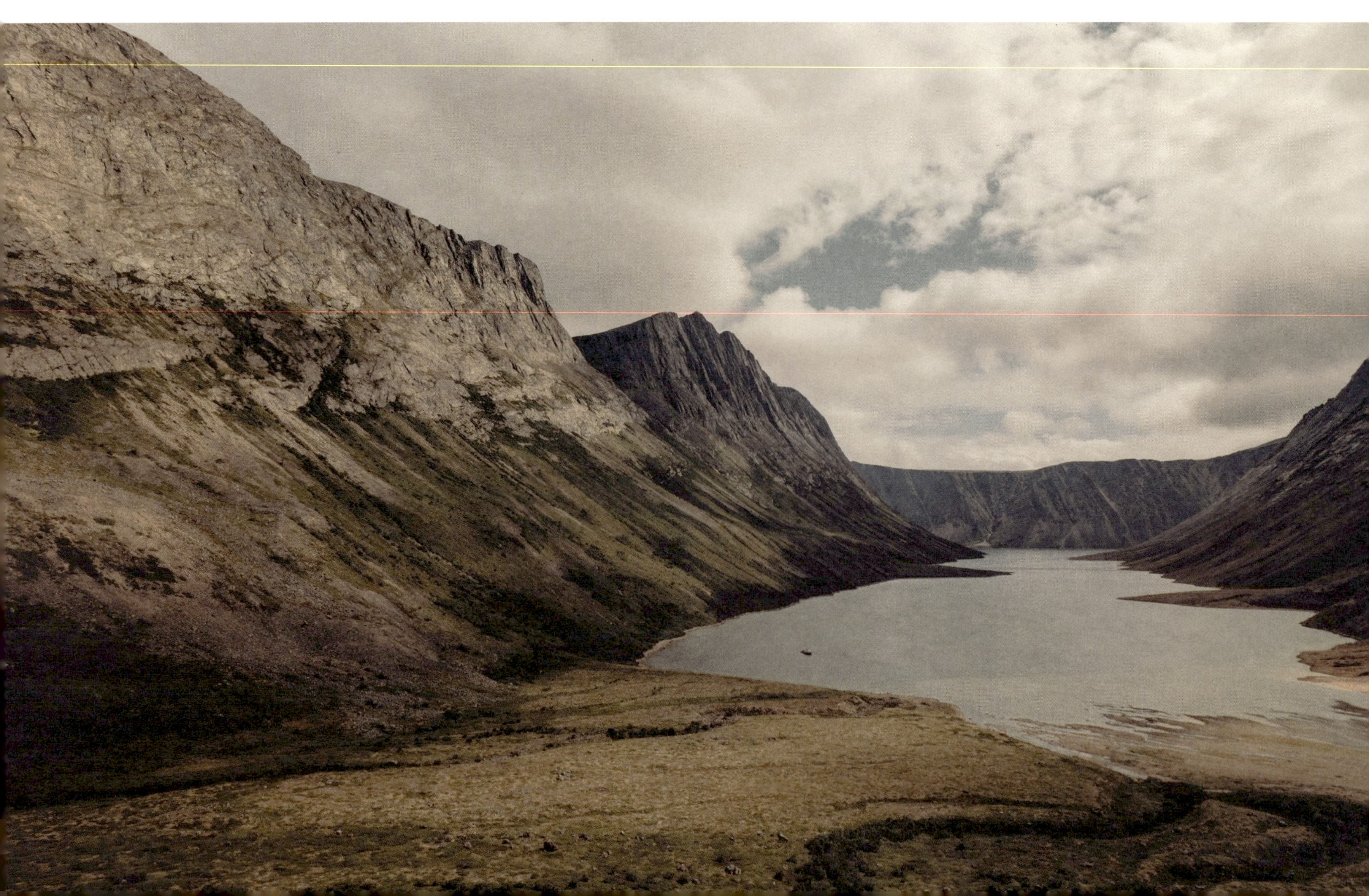

MOUNTAIN MEDICINE

I've always felt that nature is medicine. It doesn't matter if it's green spaces in big cities, a trail on the ocean's edge, or mountains like the Torngats—no matter how simple or dramatic the setting, I am always left with a renewed sense of the world around me. Nature isn't just scenery; it's a living remedy for stress, anxiety, and depression. It uplifts our mood, soothes our senses, and beckons us to engage physically. In its unscripted dance, nature's unpredictable beauty keeps our minds engaged and free from the day's clutter.

As dawn breaks, I wander through the base camp. The futuristic pods and Labrador tents fill a small area surrounded by super-charged bear fences that deter even the most curious visitors. I walk through the gate to the dock to absorb the serene ocean view. The vastness in front of me anchors my spirit, and the raw, unadorned beauty of the landscape strikes me. Such moments peel away the layers of daily fog, returning me to a state of mindfulness where inner smiles are easily found. This tranquility, a familiar and welcome guest, wraps around me. It's a connection written about in the verses of poets, validated by scientists, and sought after in our innate desire for open, untamed spaces.

Our adventure into the wild begins today. Aboard a longliner, we navigate through the majestic fjords of North Arm. The mountains, the royalty of nature, rise sharply from the ocean, reaching over a kilometre high. Polar bears and black bears dot the coastline, a reminder of the rawness of this place. Witnessing the enormity of this landscape, I'm humbled by our insignificance in this world yet filled with gratitude for experiencing such splendour.

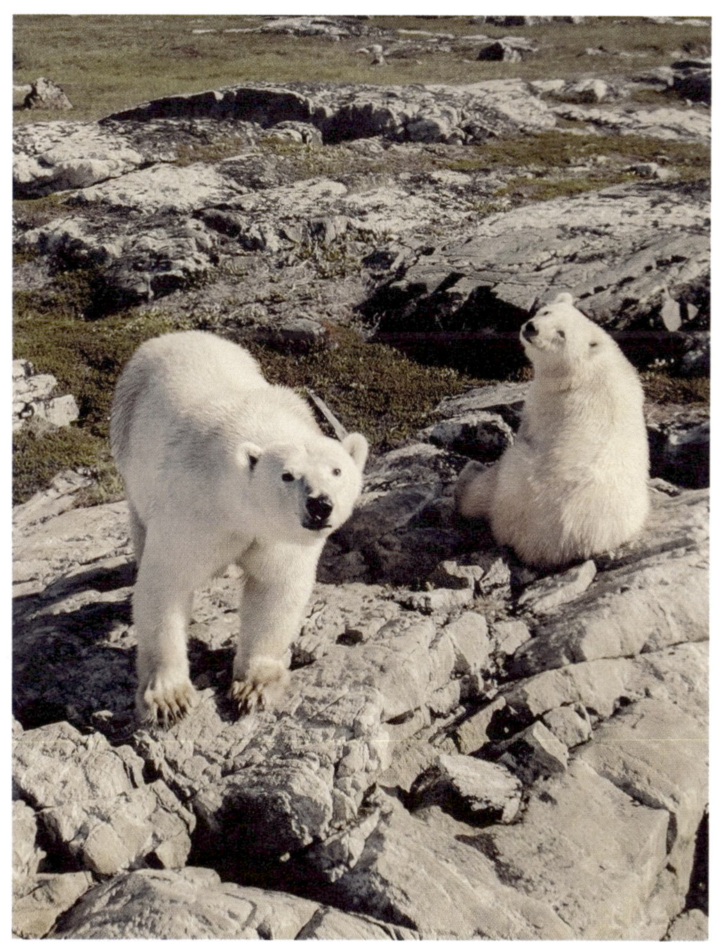

[opposite] Longliner in the Fjord
[right] Protective mother

RISKS AND REWARDS

Arriving at a remote beach, we go to board the longliner's Zodiac boat to taxi to shore but are stopped by the bear guards. They tell us to wait as one guard climbs the ladder to the upper deck while another jumps into the Zodiac with his rifle. With a rev of the engine, he swings the boat around and races to the shore.

"There . . .," one of the Inuit students points, and we see it: the slumbering polar bear, huge and dirty beige, resting on the beach about thirty metres from where we're supposed to land.

In our safety briefing, we learned the Zodiac is armed with gear designed to scare our friend from its sleep. We watch the boat pull up to the coast, slowing its engine to a low stutter. With us still on the longliner, the other bear guard, Maria, tells us to cover our ears as she fires a shot into the air to make our presence known from a distance. The bear's head lifts, awake now, but it still doesn't move.

Meanwhile, the bear guard in the Zodiac inches closer to the shore and slumbering bear, and then there's a terrific BANG! as he fires another shot into the air. The bear jumps to its feet, but the crew and I jump higher than the animal at the sound. The bear seems to be fond of its spot and fails to move any farther—that is, until a canister of whistling smoke bounces along the beach toward it. It turns and runs a safe distance, only to stare down the invisible annoyance until another canister bounces nearby. Finally, the bear has had enough and turns and runs down the beach with agility and speed. So much speed that I realize why bear guards are so essential—if a polar bear sets its sights on you, your new name is "Lunch."

Landing on the shore, our first task is to enjoy a bite to eat. The abundance of fish in this area, a lure for the polar bears, becomes our grocery store. The park rangers distribute fishing rods, and we have our catch within minutes. In a seamless display of wilderness expertise, our guides set up a fire. The sizzling of bright orange char on the heated rocks, the preparation of bannock bread by the Inuit elders, and the picturesque scene of my companions fishing against a backdrop of immense cliffs is too perfect to describe. The sheer scale of the mountains, dwarfing even the grandeur of skyscrapers, challenges me to comprehend the magnificence surrounding us. In this moment, clarity and presence envelop me, and the world feels impossibly serene and perfect.

But life's unpredictability soon disrupts our peace. A cry for help shatters the quiet, and I see Braeden bent over and yelling. He is struggling with a fishing lure gone awry, causing a chaotic blend of blood and metal. The swift response of our expedition nurse, coupled with Braeden's predicament, highlights our vulnerability even in leisurely moments.

As Braeden's ordeal with the fishing hook unfolds, I'm struck by how swiftly a state of mind can shift from tranquility to urgency. There is a delicate equilibrium we maintain between adventure and safety. Yet, as the immediate crisis subsides, the rhythmic sounds of the waves and the inviting aroma of the char on the fire gently guide us back to the moment. The vastness of the landscape reassures us, and we realign with our surroundings. Bandaged but undeterred, Braeden, ever the creative spirit, readies his camera, his enthusiasm undiminished.

[opposite] Waterfall on route to the glacier lake

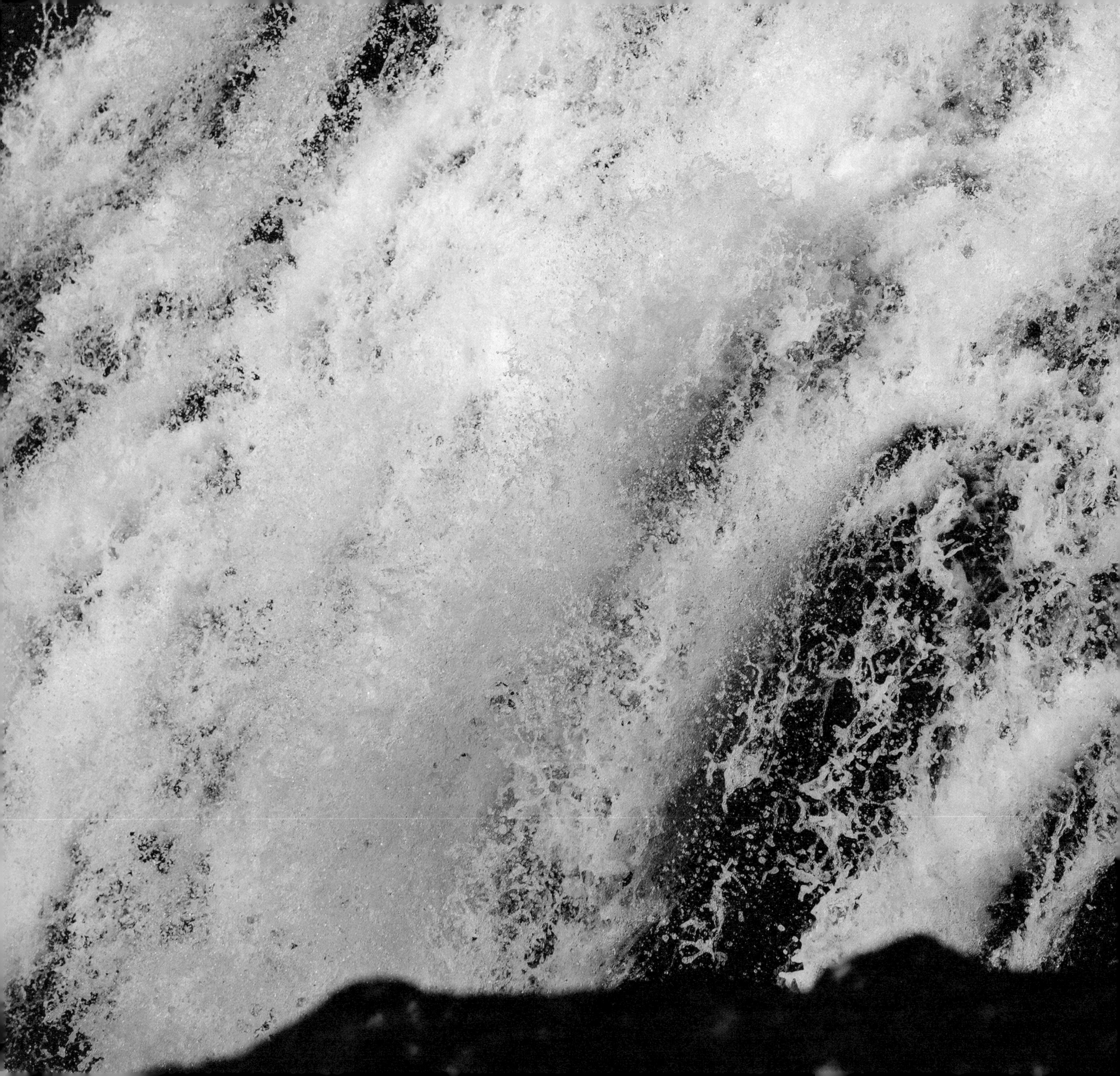

SHINING LIGHT ON NATURE'S GIFTS

We are headed inland to a place I have only dreamed of seeing—a stunning glacier lake nestled between the massive cliffs accompanying the fjord. We climb steadily upward, finding waterfalls with ice-cold water that refreshes as we trudge through the brush and flies. Before long, we summit a hill to discover our destination. The lake reflects the sky with a brilliant blue shine, revealing a stark dichotomy in the surrounding landscape. The mountains on one side are green from sun exposure, while the other side is a rusty orange of shaded barren rock and soil.

The contrast underscores how far north we are, and it reminds me of how our health can mirror that desolate mountain face when hidden from the sun and shrouded in darkness. That darkness, whether figurative or real, stifles our growth and wilts our form. Our bodies and minds thrive in nature, much like that green slope. Nature eases the strain on our systems and the pressure in our bodies; it calms our hearts and releases molecules that restore and heal. It counteracts the glow of screens and the sound of machines that are all too common in our daily lives. We grow in green spaces like the plants that keep us company in nature.

I walk in the sun and am restored. For many, good health can seem like a mountain—imposing, impassable, and impossible. Examining our health is like finding our bearings. With reflection, we may realize we are descending toward a shaded face, but with a simple turn, we start to climb back up to a place where we can thrive. As we embark on our journey toward our goals, particularly those related to our health, we often confront seemingly insurmountable obstacles. Yet, as we draw closer, it becomes evident that what we initially perceive as a towering mountain is merely a hill.

My journey to the North and those majestic cliffs emphasizes the importance of taking time to think, move, and breathe. This place of spirits has sent many messengers to visit me. It reminds me of nature's power in the form of polar bears and incredible cliffs; it sends adversity and demands respect for the ecosystem and food chain; it imbues me with a feeling of appreciation for a culture I knew very little about.

It's a beautiful awakening.

We steam home, and our evening finishes with an invitation to compete in the Inuit games. Leg wrestling, high kicks, and feats of strength unite our camp of people in friendly competition. I look around and see that the group of people who arrived as strangers are now communing as one, appreciating, respecting, and relating.

It's a connection forged by our time together in nature.

Nature is an intrinsic part of our being, resonating within us in a deeply visceral way. It connects us to our minds and our bodies. The awe-inspiring mountains of the North serve as a powerful metaphor that we can overcome the most daunting of obstacles—even those that deceive us into forgetting the beauty of the world around us.

GETTING HIGH ON NATURE

Getting high on nature might be the best way to escape modern life's day-to-day stresses. Outdoor environments offer a range of benefits for both physical and mental health. From our experience in the Torngat Mountains, we've discovered several essential ways that nature is the best medicine:

ACTIVITY CLIMBS: Mountains are great for hiking, climbing, and other physical activities.

HEART BEATS: Altitude improves cardiovascular health by increasing lung capacity and blood oxygen levels.

HIGHER PERSPECTIVES: A mountain setting will reduce symptoms of stress and anxiety and improve overall mental well-being.

EN"LIGHT"ENMENT: The abundance of light above the clouds regulates circadian rhythms and promotes healthy sleep patterns.

ELEMENTAL HEALTH: Nature improves our immune system by exposing us to fresh air and a clean environment.

ELEVATED BONDING: Connecting with others is easier without the distractions of daily life and modern technology. We can foster deeper bonds with those around us.

PEAK CREATIVITY: Natural expanses like mountain ranges increase creativity and problem-solving abilities.

TAKE ACTION IN NATURE

Follow these simple rules to make the most out of your bond with the natural world:

TAKE A DAILY STROLL: Devote at least thirty minutes daily to wander through a natural setting, be it a park, woodland, or along the water's edge. This simple act will help you forge a connection with nature and alleviate stress.

CULTIVATE MINDFULNESS IN NATURE: Seek out a serene outdoor spot, settle into a comfortable position, and concentrate on your breathing for a few moments. Allow yourself to absorb the sounds, sights, and fragrances around you without judgment.

INVITE THE OUTSIDE IN: Introduce plants to your home and work environments to enhance indoor air quality and establish a soothing atmosphere.

UNPLUG FROM THE DIGITAL WORLD: Carve out time daily to disconnect from screens and devices. Utilize this opportunity to engage with your environment and the natural world.

EXPLORE NATURE IN YOUR COMMUNITY: Visit local parks, nature preserves, or botanical gardens.

JOIN A NATURE-ORIENTED GROUP OR CLUB: Socialize with those who share your appreciation for nature. Participate in group hikes, birdwatching excursions, or nature photography sessions to nurture your connection to the natural world and your social circle.

OUR HEALTH SHERPAS

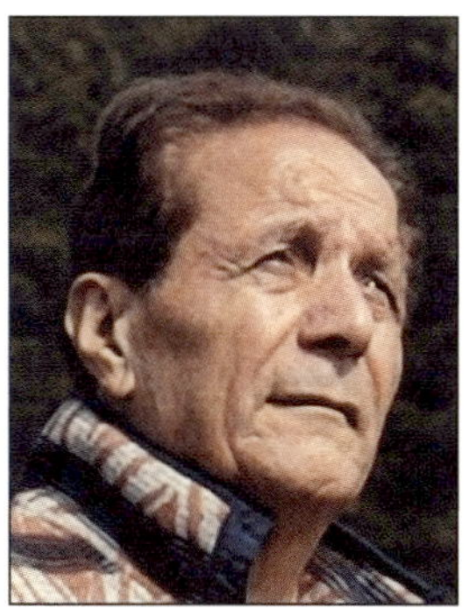

DR. HASSAN KHALILI: Doc believes that one of the best treatments for the challenges to our mental health is all around us. "Nature gives it to us, the trees, water—you don't have to go too far" to benefit from nature if you live in a place like Newfoundland and Labrador. But if you want to go further, his advice is to take a mental picture and visit your goal regularly so achieving it will seem familiar and attainable. If that goal is travel, Doc suggests prioritizing nature and immersing yourself fully so you can reconnect in what we sometimes forget is our natural habitat.

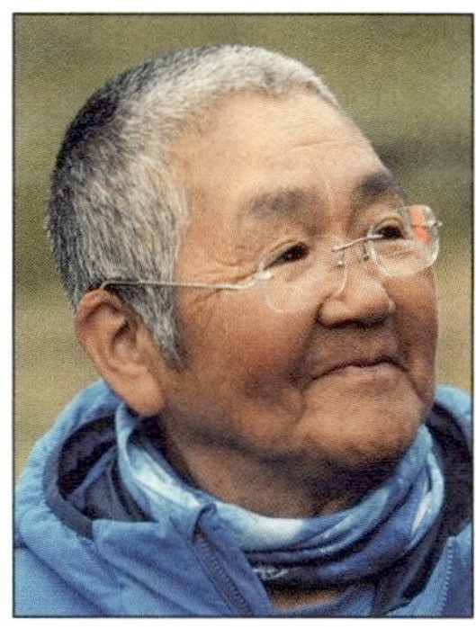

MARIA MERKURATSUK: Maria was one of our bear guards and storytellers on our Torngat adventure. She grew up on the land and uses it to teach the next generation in her community. She is a knowledge holder and mentor whose life has been shaped by the North. For all her adventures, hunts, and history, she, like so many others who have spent time in this beautiful land, can't describe it with words. That is something she says people have to see and experience for themselves.

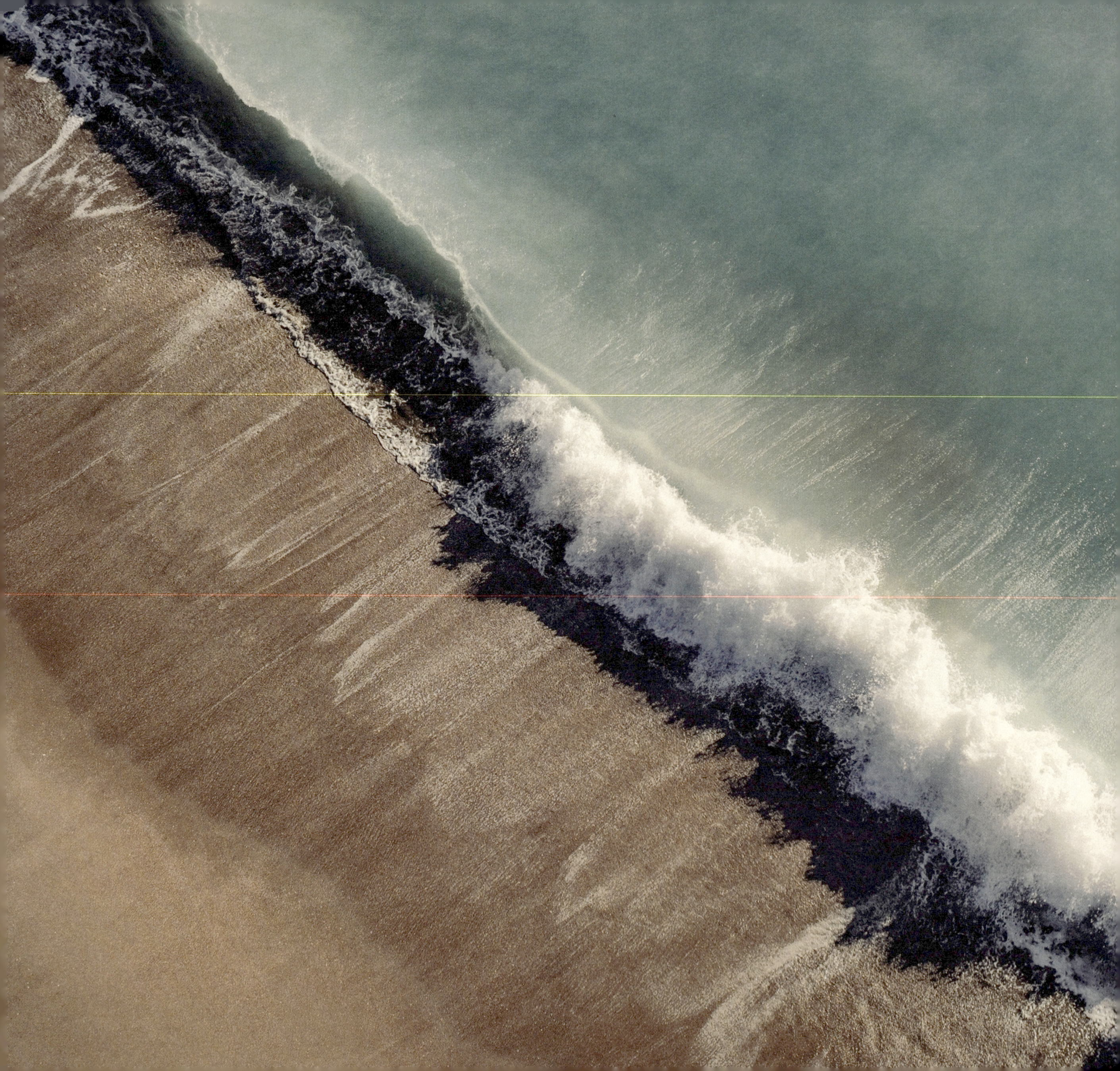

2

WAVES OF HEALING

On New Zealand's rugged coastline, I rediscover the therapeutic essence of water, a natural extension of my lifelong connection to this elemental force. In a world rife with stress and demands, my interactions with New Zealand's waters offer a window into a universal remedy for the soul.

AN UNLIKELY COMPANION

In the heart of the North Atlantic, where the frigid winds howl and wild waves crash against our rocky shores, an unlikely sanctuary calls to me.

In the middle of winter, the water is an icy adversary that holds a secret worth braving the biting cold. As I paddle out on my surfboard from the shore, freezing spray hits my face. My heart pounds with anticipation as I navigate the turbulent sea, motivated by an unexplainable desire to immerse myself in its depths.

The waves rise and fall with hypnotic rhythm. I watch each crest appear on the horizon, analyzing where the face will crumble and froth into a white-water barrier. Far from the safety of the shore, I find myself suspended in the moment as the approaching wave looms. Filling my lungs with air, I dive beneath the surface, surrendering to the water's heavy surge.

Beneath the waves lies a silent realm where time loses its grip and thoughts disperse. The salt water stings my half-open eyes, and I see the surface drawing near as a wave passes overhead. Emerging, I gasp for a new breath. The piercing air bites my face, awakening every nerve and reminding me that I'm alive.

Along the coast, a rocky cliffside towers. It offers respite from the relentless winds. Free from the gale's annoyance, the ocean transforms into a glassy trail of corduroy waves, inviting me to play with the rhythm of the sea.

My purpose here transcends the pursuit of catching waves. It is the water itself, this elemental force, that serves as my escape. In its embrace, no matter how numbing the chill, I find peace—a remedy for life's daily stresses. In the vastness of the ocean, I have discovered a meditation unlike any other, a source of healing that only the ocean can provide me.

Throughout my life, I've enjoyed a deep connection with water. Born next to the Great Lakes, raised in a town divided by a river, and spending childhood summers between our backyard pool and my grandparents' cabin by a fishing river, I've always considered being close to water an integral part of my existence. Even during my spare time while I worked in the United States, I would kayak in the waters of the Long Island Sound.

Now, I live less than 100 metres from the ocean. I find comfort and tranquility knowing it is in my backyard. I proposed to my wife by the ocean, have spent many weekends camping at the ocean's edge, and sought consolation on the coast during the challenging times of the pandemic. Reflecting on these experiences, I realize that water has always held an inexplicable power to wash away my worries and bring me a deep sense of calm. It is this personal connection that fuels my curiosity and pushes me to embark on a search, eager to explore whether this intimate bond with water is a universal experience.

[previous page] The blue mind
[opposite] Ribbons of swell at sunset in Taranaki

THE LONG WAY AROUND

My journey leads me to the far reaches of the world, where unfamiliar constellations dot the sky and volcanoes have shaped an island paradise that the Māori people call home. Guided by a trail of clues, as if I were tracking a ship's wake, I connect with Hayden, my newfound friend and water man. He shares his love for the ocean, liberating others—even if only momentarily—from the grasp of their thoughts through his surf therapy program known as Restoke. It's a fitting name (especially if you understand surfing terminology) that renews the spirits and ignites the flame of resilience in individuals who are overcoming life's challenges.

My crew and I have come to New Zealand—an island nation almost diametrically opposed on the globe from my own island home—to learn more about the connection between water and well-being,

Leaving Auckland, we wind along roads for hours through lush green mountains until the setting sun paints a breathtaking canvas above. Leaving the high peaks and dropping to the coast, we park our vehicle on the roadside as we are greeted by an incredible sight. The sky blushes shades of scarlet, and the imposing peak of the Mount Taranaki volcano commands the horizon. The sea stretches out forever in front of us and is adorned with ribbons of a western swell. The ocean breeze, gentle and warm, carries the unmistakable scent of salt water, reminding me of home. With camera in hand, Braeden deftly leaps over a wire fence, determined to capture the skyline as we wade through waist-high grass. This moment marks the culmination of a long journey to what the locals affectionately call "Taradise." Without the need for explanation, I understand why it bears such a fitting name.

We settle into our small beach house for the night after our long voyage.

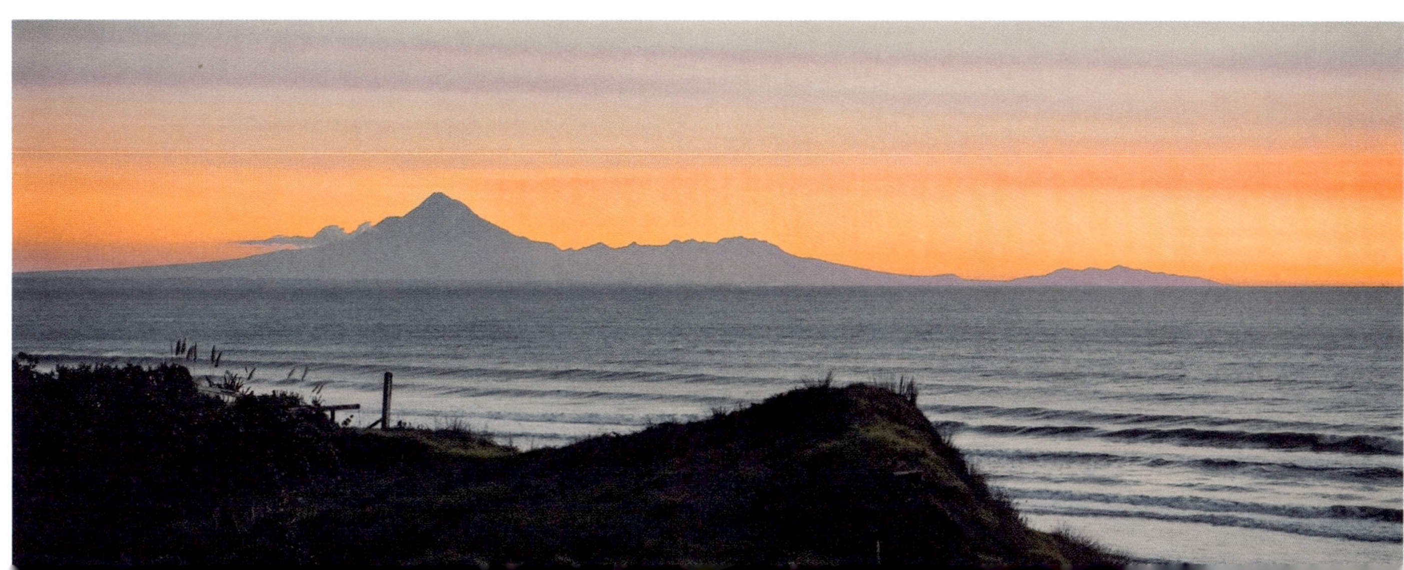

RESTOKED

Our day begins with a short drive from New Plymouth to a local surf break, where we are warmly welcomed by our new friends at a beach house filled with vibrant blue foam boards and beaming faces. As I embrace Hayden, I feel a sense of shared familiarity, and he introduces me to his co-workers and the participants of his inspiring program. Restoke, a surf therapy program unlike any other, merges the power of nature and traditional therapy to create a unique approach to healing.

Restoke's philosophy combines the exhilaration of surfing with one-on-one counselling, support, and therapeutic practices both in and out of the water. Participants are chosen through a competitive application process in which they express why they believe water and surfing can unlock their hidden potential.

By intertwining physical activity, the natural environment, and evidence-based therapy techniques, Restoke offers a comprehensive and individualized approach to supporting mental and emotional well-being.

The program's success has earned it international recognition, yet Restoke remains grounded in its mission to help one person at a time. It values the restorative power of the ocean and is dedicated to fostering growth, resilience, and self-discovery. Through Restoke, Hayden and his team encourage participants to confront their challenges head-on, providing a safe and supportive space where the healing qualities of water can be harnessed to their fullest potential.

Among Hayden's team is Josie, the vibrant van-dwelling "hype girl" whose infectious enthusiasm sets the tone for the day. Her effervescent spirit and boundless energy inspire those around her, creating an atmosphere of excitement and motivation. Whether it's cheering on fellow surfers or encouraging others to step out of their comfort zones, Josie's presence embodies the transformative power of the ocean. She shares her own journey of overcoming personal challenges through the healing embrace of the waves, serving as an example of hope and encouragement for others seeking healing through the Restoke program.

Nigel, another member of the team, possesses a natural ability to support and uplift others. Effortlessly, he finds deep fulfillment in the simplest of tasks during each session. Nigel mingles with the participants as a peer. He laughs with them and shares the surf conditions for the day. I overhear him reassuring a nervous "restoker" that he will provide a push to help them catch waves in the session so they can be guaranteed to have fun. Nigel's presence is one of ease and compassion, fostering a sense of community and acceptance within the group. His laid-back approach seems to create a safe space where healing and personal growth can flourish.

Hayden is tall and lanky, with broad shoulders built through surfing, and bleach-blond hair, a testament to hours in the sun. His eyes are as blue as the ocean, welcoming you in with an understanding softness. As I observe Hayden interacting with the participants, his gentle nature and innate talent for connection become evident. Like a reef breaking the energy of waves, his tranquil demeanour creates a calm and nurturing environment. Hayden chats with each participant, his genuine interest evident in his mannerisms and questions. It is clear that he's invested in these individuals, hustling about to grab wetsuits, boards, wax, and whatever his participants need. It is his nature.

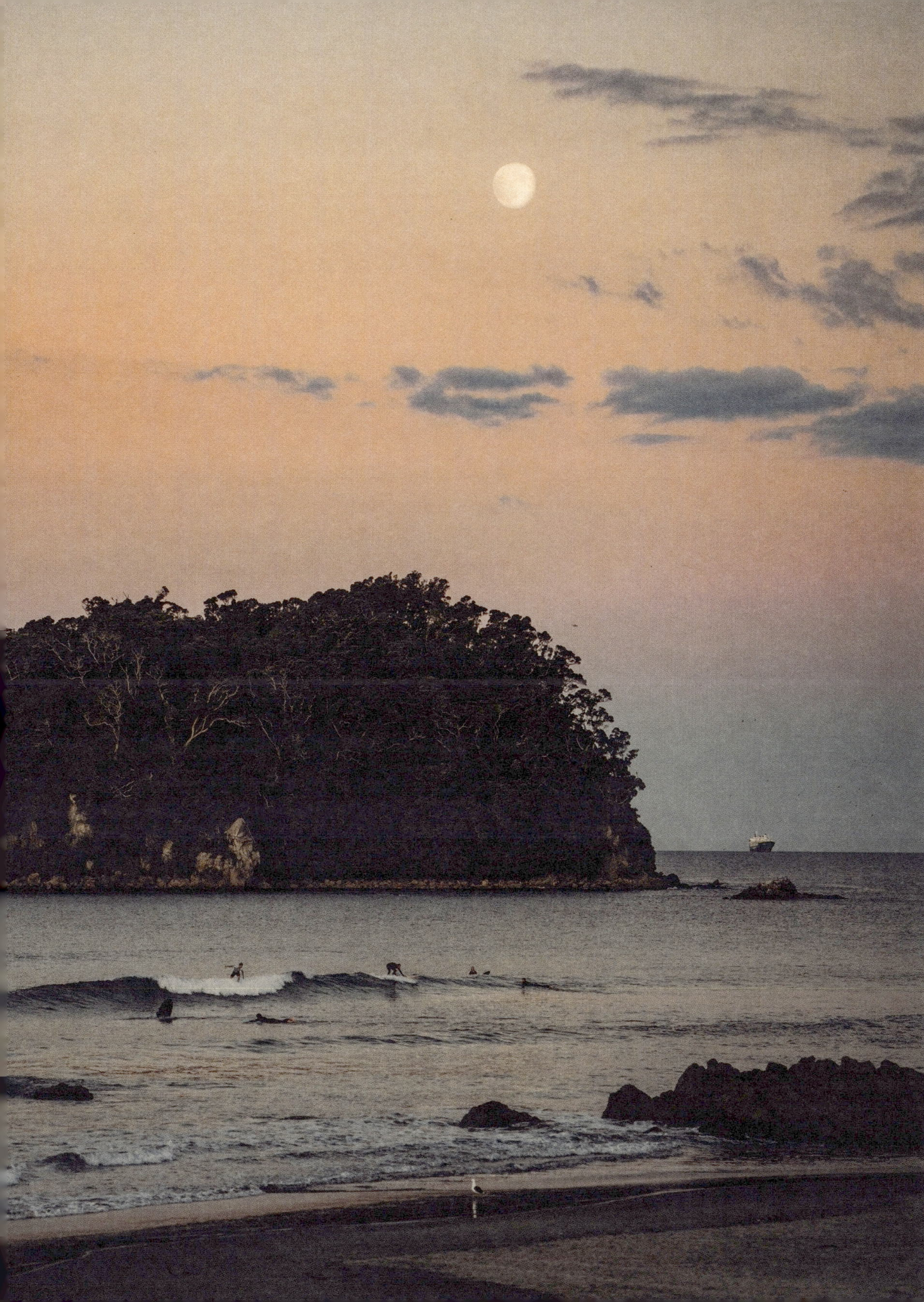

He is warm and consoling; whether through a gentle pat on the back or a big hug during a proud moment, he is unapologetically kind.

The program participants represent a diverse variety of life experiences and narratives, each finding their own unique path to healing through water. Hayden introduces me to three program participants who each represent a different struggle in mental health and illustrate the complexity that comes with overcoming one's own challenges.

Surfing under the moon

VULNERABILITY, SELF-WORTH, AND RESURGENCE

I meet Nick, an introspective twenty-something with a bold new-school mullet, who has embarked on a courageous journey of rediscovery. Despite being a former competitive surfer, he lost his passion for both the water and life itself. Now a construction worker, Nick hesitated to seek help, fearing judgment from his co-workers in an industry that often emphasizes a stereotypical view of masculinity and stability. But being in the presence of fellow program participants who were experiencing the wonders of the ocean for the first time reignited Nick's love for the water—and that love became a powerful catalyst for his personal transformation.

Despite facing the obstacle of a broken ankle, he warmly greeted us with his guitar in hand, serenading his fellow group members as they prepared to don their wetsuits. Nick and Hayden met through the close-knit surf community in their area. Aware of Hayden's program, Nick approached him after a joint surf session, saying, "Bro, I really need help; I can't find anyone to talk to, and I need a shake-up." Since completing the program, Nick has remained involved, offering peer support to others. Through his personal journey of reflection and surrender, Nick came to a profound realization—self-protectionism was an ineffective shield against depression. With the support of the ocean and the community surrounding him, he revived relationships, purpose, and an evolved sense of self.

Nick's story reflects the fears and struggles that countless individuals who face mental health challenges encounter. The pressure to maintain an outward facade of strength and the reluctance to admit the need for help are familiar burdens. However, Nick's journey of acknowledging his vulnerabilities and actively seeking support exemplifies courage. By openly sharing his story, Nick illuminates the importance of addressing mental health and fostering open conversations about emotional well-being. His experience also reminds us that the fear of vulnerability often stems from our own insecurities rather than the judgments of those around us. Ultimately, Nick's story is a powerful reminder that true strength lies in embracing our struggles, so we can find healing and embark on a path that serves us.

Moana now floats into our presence. Aptly named after the Māori word for ocean, she emanates a spiritual depth derived from her heritage and a lifetime of exploration. As a mother of two children, she understands that the struggles she has faced can have a profound impact on her role as a parent. Initially, Moana held reservations about joining the program, feeling undeserving and believing that it should be reserved for others who may need it more. She carried a sense of guilt, doubting whether she should take the opportunity available to her.

Upon joining Restoke, Moana discovered that participating in the program was the most powerful thing she had ever done for herself. She found peace in sitting beyond the break, embracing the serene space that exists before the crashing waves. I witness this ritual as the session begins. With some help from

Hayden, she navigates the white water to appear behind a set of waves, peacefully floating and observing. Through the lens of the ocean, Moana has begun to see the world in a new light, gaining a unique perspective that brings her intense harmony. The healing power of the ocean has become undeniable to her, and she has developed a new appreciation for the freedom she has attained through her time connecting with her namesake.

Moana's experience within the Restoke program resonates with the team, including Hayden, who admires her willingness to confront her own self-doubts and recognizes the importance of prioritizing her well-being, which ultimately makes her more available to those around her—including her children.

And then I meet Yasmine, a young and reserved individual who carries the weight of the challenges she faces each day. Coming of age during the pandemic, she bears a hesitancy that speaks to the overwhelming impact it has had on her life. In a moment of vulnerability, Yasmine discloses that her decision to participate in the Restoke program is driven by a deep desire to connect with her father, a surfer who battled mental health issues and tragically ended his life when she was only six years old. Hayden, an accomplished surfer himself, struck her as the kind of mentor her late father would have endorsed. She entrusted him with teaching her the sport and guiding her through her personal challenges.

With courage, Yasmine shares her personal growth and the newfound connection she has forged with the ocean. She navigates the waves with determination, channelling her emotions into each stroke and finding strength in the sea. In the quietude of the ocean's embrace, she finds a sense of accomplishment in learning to surf that allows her to heal the wounds left by her father's absence. As we speak, she gazes fondly over the waves. Her eyes well up with tears that reflect both sorrow and optimism, and she quietly expresses her hope that her father would be proud of the person she has become.

Jared Dixon

Yasmine's story serves as a poignant reminder of the lasting impact of loss and the profound ways in which the ocean can aid in the healing process. By immersing herself in the restorative embrace of the water, Yasmine finds a connection to her father, writing a new story of their relationship and allowing him to guide her to healing. Through this growth, she has discovered her own strength, resilience, and capacity, honouring her father's memory by cherishing the best parts of him within herself.

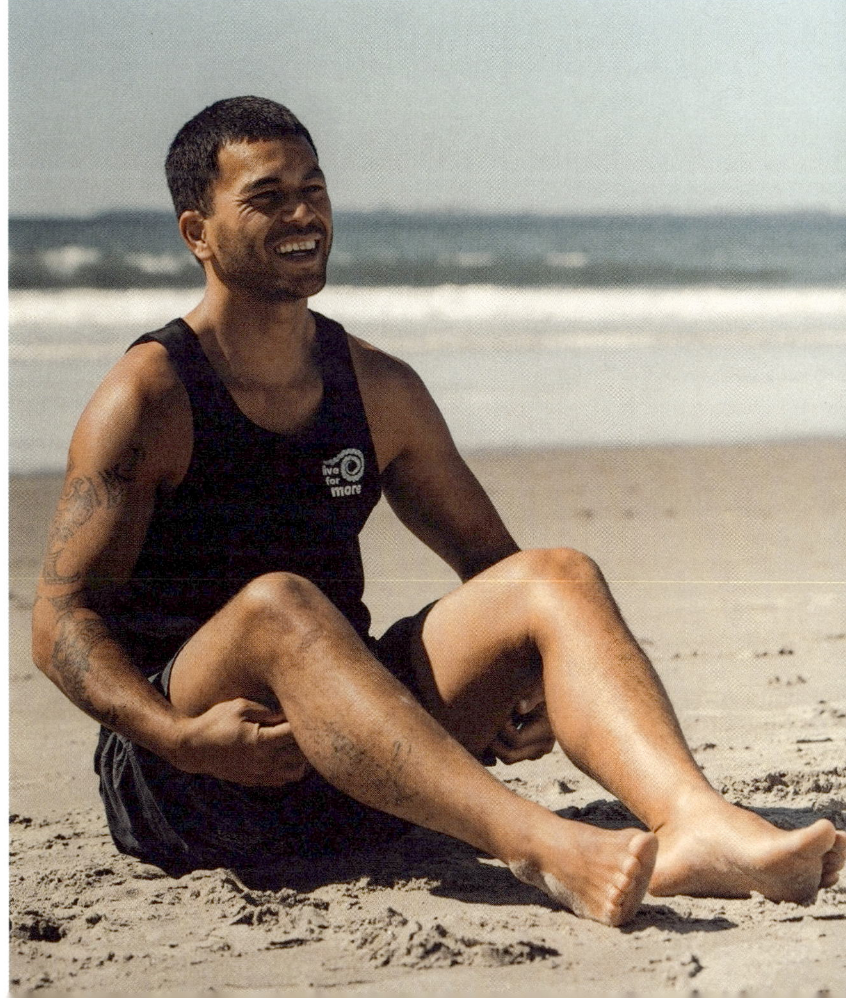

EBB AND FLOW

With anticipation, I slip into my wetsuit and stretch, a ritual that ignites the feeling of being a first-time surfer once more. The innocence of the moment is not lost on me, offering a fresh perspective that contrasts with the exhilaration and urgency of entering cold northern waters. As I step into the warm embrace of the ocean, the waves crash and splash against my giant floaty surfboard, which resonates deep within me. I smile.

There is a beautiful simplicity to our gathering. We laugh and paddle through the gentle waves. Each stroke propels us forward, synchronized in our efforts as we try for waves in turn. Cheering for a good attempt fills the air, not only for the accomplishment of catching a wave but also for the collective energy and joy that permeates the experience. The goal of riding a wave becomes secondary, if not inconsequential, giving way to fun as we exist for a time in the present moment.

Here, on the opposite side of the world, I am surprised by an overwhelming sense of belonging. The ocean, the eternal conduit that connects our two homes, transcends the boundaries of geography. It becomes a universal entity, embracing us all with its energy and healing power. The water splashes my face, this time a gentle touch, but it awakens my senses like the frigid waters back home. It reminds me it is the same mindful ally and is absolutely essential.

As I ride the waves on my bright blue board, surrendering to their ebb and flow, I feel the "stoke" of even the tiniest rides. It's why the program is so aptly named. The water becomes our playground, and I'm filled with the exhilarating joy of a child with new friends. This feeling of stoke, born from our love of surf and the thrill that comes from doing what excites and inspires us, permeates every moment of this experience. It's a reminder to embrace our passions, rediscover our inner fire, and find happiness in the simplest of acts.

In this moment, I recognize that the healing influence of water extends beyond its physical properties. It holds the capacity to cleanse our souls, to wash away the weight of the world and leave us renewed. The ocean is a sanctuary, a space where camaraderie, laughter, and healing can intertwine.

Here, in the embrace of the universal entity that is the ocean, I discover a sense of wholeness and a deep understanding that we are all connected by the miracle of water.

[opposite] The Taranaki volcano

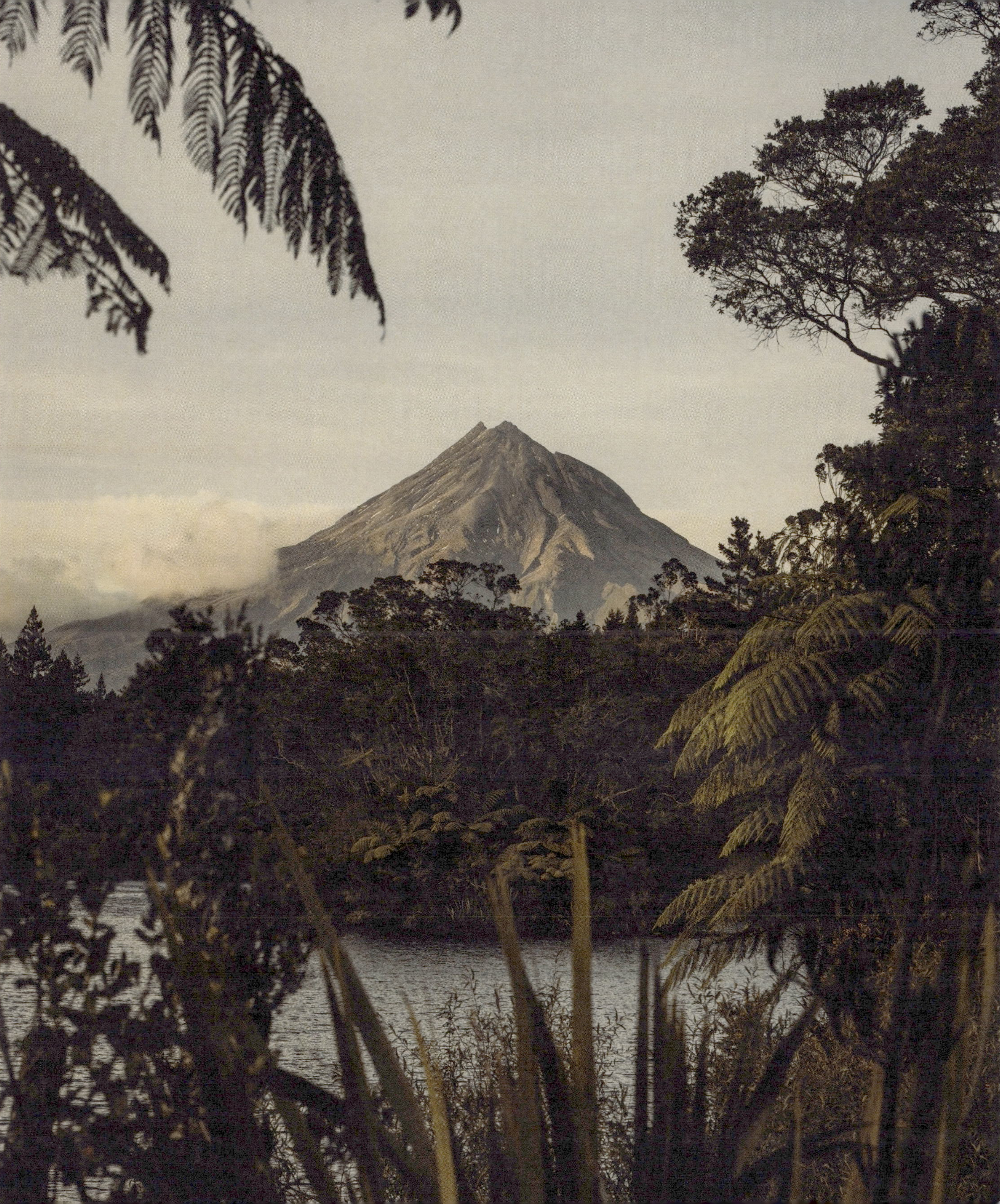

HEALING WATERS: ENHANCING MIND AND BODY THROUGH WATER

The following action items demonstrate how water, in its various forms and environments, has the power to heal and improve our well-being both physically and mentally. By incorporating these practices into your life, you can prioritize and enjoy the healing and beneficial effects of water, promoting your overall health and well-being.

WATER CALMS: Water has a soothing effect on the mind and body, promoting relaxation and reducing stress levels. Set aside time each day for a calming water ritual, such as taking a soothing bath, enjoying a hot shower, or practising mindfulness near a water source like a fountain or waterfall. Use this dedicated time to relax, reflect, and let go of daily stresses.

WATER HEALS: Water supports physical fitness and overall health, and water therapy, such as hydrotherapy or aquatic exercise, can alleviate pain and promote physical healing. The buoyancy of water reduces the impact on joints and muscles, making it an ideal environment for rehabilitation or for those with joint pain or injury. Incorporate water-based activities into your fitness routine, such as swimming, kayaking, paddleboarding, or even walking and hiking along the beach or coastline.

WATER MOVES: Being near bodies of water, such as lakes, rivers, or the ocean, has been linked to improved mental health and well-being. The calming effect of the sound of water, such as waves crashing or a babbling brook, combined with the beauty of nature, has a therapeutic effect on the brain, helping to reduce the symptoms of depression and mental fatigue and promote mindfulness and increase feelings of happiness of serenity. Make an effort to seek out natural bodies of water. Plan outings to these locations for picnics or walks, or simply to enjoy the calming sights and sounds of the water. If you can't get to a natural body of water, buy a small fountain for your home, or even download an app that offers the soothing sound of waves, brooks, or rain.

OUR WATER GUIDES

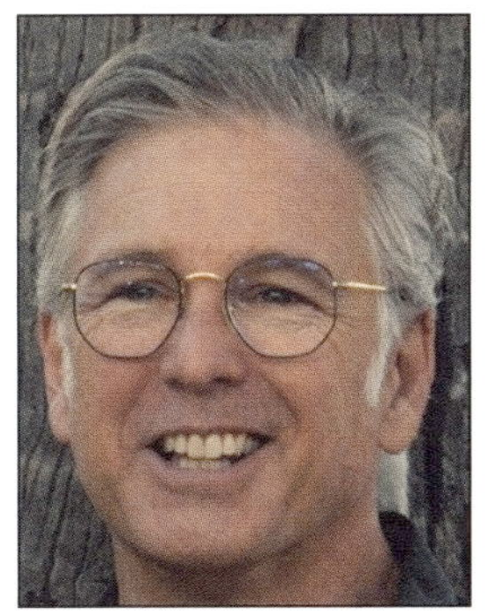

DR. WALLACE J. NICHOLS: On an earlier trip to explore the power of water in Honolulu, Hawaii, I had the privilege of diving deep into the subject with Dr. Wallace J. Nichols, a renowned expert on the healing power of water. Dr. Nichols, *The New York Times* bestselling author of *Blue Mind*, has dedicated his work to uncovering the profound effects of being in, near, or around water on our well-being. Through his research, he has demonstrated that water has a significant positive impact on our health. Dr. Nichols promotes the concept of "Bluescriptions," encouraging individuals to develop intentional habits that involve water, recognizing its therapeutic potential. His insights have reshaped our understanding of the connection between water and our overall well-being, inspiring us to embrace the healing influence of water in our lives.

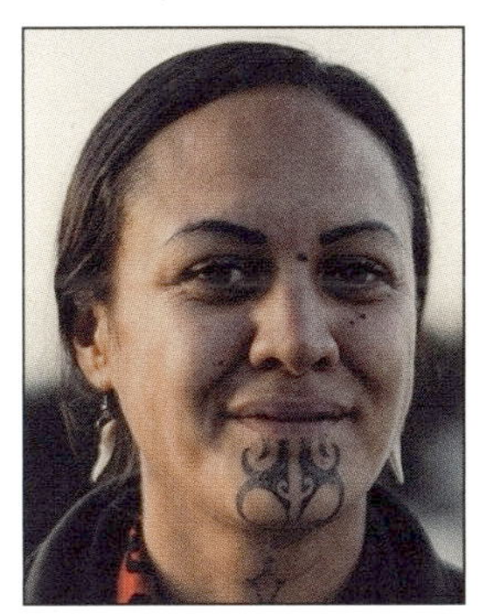

MORGAN TE HURIHANGANUI: En route to Restoke while in New Zealand, we stopped in at the Te Puia thermal geysers and had the privilege of being guided by Morgan, a sixth-generation Māori knowledge holder. She shared with us the cultural and spiritual importance of water in Māori traditions. Water is intricately woven into their language, ceremonies, and daily lives. Through a deeply personal experience, Morgan revealed how immersing herself in the geyser spray provided a profound connection to her late husband, as they shared a deep bond with the thermal pools. Following a devastating loss in her family, waters from her home helped her find solace and reconnect with cherished memories. Through her story, we learned that water, or wai in Māori, is not just vital for physical health but also essential for the overall well-being and spiritual nourishment of the Māori people.

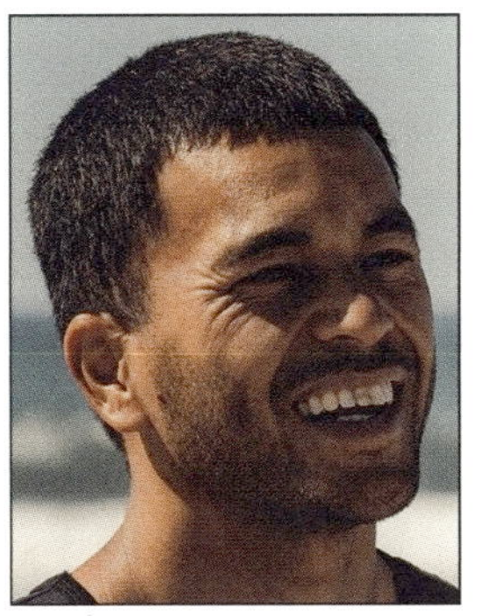

JARED DIXON: I met Jared during my travels in New Zealand and witnessed the transformative power that being in or around water can have on an individual. When Jared's life took a challenging turn, leading to encounters with the law and time spent in jail, he recognized the need for change. He embraced a new path through the Live for More surf therapy program. The power of the ocean had a profound impact on him, altering the course of his life. Drawing from his deep cultural connection as a Māori, he found healing and personal growth in ways that the formal systems of society had failed to provide. Inspired by his own journey, Jared now serves as a mentor for new students and plays an integral role in running the Live for More program. Through his experiences, Jared learned to live for more, discovering the incredible potential for healing and transformation that lies within the embrace of the ocean.

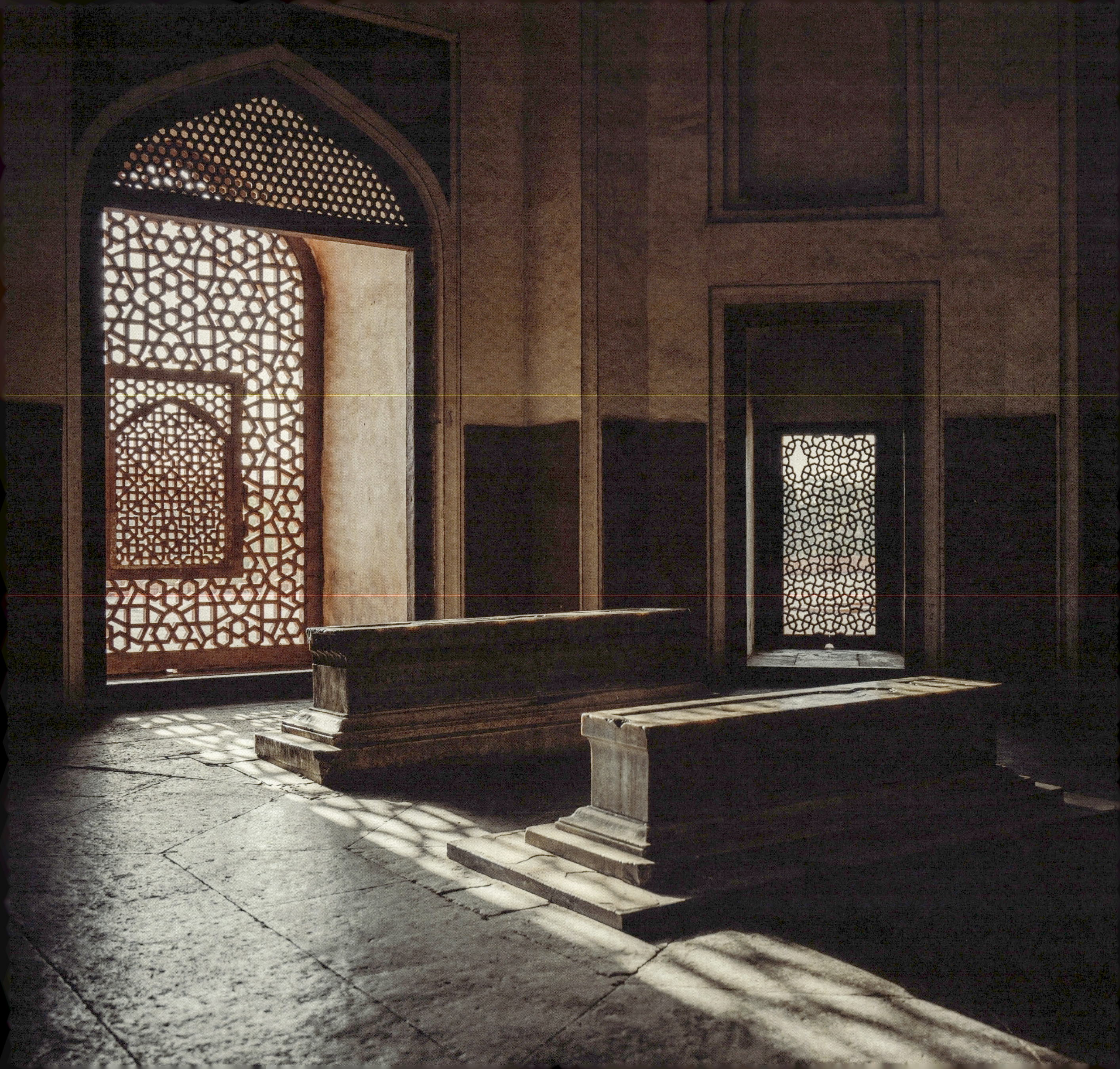

ORDER WITHIN CHAOS

Delhi encompasses a captivating blend of chaos and spirituality that challenges and enlightens the soul. As I journey through its bustling streets and meet its people, I find an unexpected balance that resonates long after I leave. In a world speeding toward complexity, Delhi stands as a paradoxical guide to internal harmony. The city teaches that even amidst external chaos, inner peace is not just possible but transformative.

THE DUALITIES OF DELHI

As the day breaks, the scorching sun rises over a hazy skyline. Rays of golden light pierce through the blinds of my hotel room, prying my eyes open. The crew and I arrived in New Delhi at midnight after a long journey from New Zealand. Thanks to the assistance of the Indian Embassy in Canada, our passage through customs was smooth and I've been able to score a few hours of sleep.

I look out over the expressway, where vehicles dance across highway lines and traffic flows with noisy urgency. Today, our journey takes us into that commotion as we set out to explore Old Delhi. Leaving the modern, hotel-packed Aerocity district, a hub for tourists and business travellers, we make our way to the city's historical heart. To reach it, we drive along the highway until it plunges into an underground tunnel. This passageway feels like a stark divide between two worlds: on one side a city steeped in Western luxury and conveniences, and on the other, a place where life unfolds with tangible authentic intensity.

Emerging into the crowded streets, I struggle to absorb the scene before me. Stunted buildings, dusty storefronts, and a swarm of nameless faces squeeze our accustomed personal space to nothing. We meander through the labyrinth of streets, cameras in hand, our attention pulled in every direction. The sensory overload is challenging. Food vendors prepare naan bread and curries, spice traders bargain energetically, and tuk-tuks maneuver through impossibly small spaces like expert pilots. It's a perpetual sea of activity, a way of life vastly different from the way we prioritize personal space in the West. Yet, within the chaos, India discovers its own order and peace of mind. My goal is to understand this remarkable equilibrium.

Navigating through the alleys, we eventually arrive at a street adorned with orange flags, signalling the entrance to a bustling gurdwara, a white temple frequented by Sikhs. Observing the rituals of removing our shoes, wrapping our hair, and washing our feet, we step inside. There are musicians playing unfamiliar instruments, which fill the temple with melodic verses known as kirtan. We sit among the devotees, taking in the sights and sounds of this spiritual spectacle. After some time, we exit through the back of the temple and encounter a large pool of water where people bathe, creating a communal courtyard of cleansing. Families seek respite from the midday sun, finding solace under stone overhangs. As we leave, a sweet dough called Karah Parshad is given to us as a token of gratitude. Unwrapping our hair and collecting our shoes, we rejoin the throng of visitors and are carried by the crowd to our next destination.

From there, our journey leads us to a towering mosque just a short distance away. The intricate architecture and towering minarets reach toward the sky with a simplistic grandeur. Ascending the steps, we join the stream of visitors, respectfully removing our shoes before entering. The sprawling courtyard welcomes worshipers from all walks of life, offering a sanctuary for prayer and reflection. Inside, the vast expanse reveals a serene and sacred space designed with graceful arches.

A tradition of faith resonates through this community that is not bounded by specific religion.

Not far from the mosque, we arrive at a colourful square with pillars and towers, leading to a Hindu temple. Our guide speaks with a vendor and hands me a box of sweets along with some simple instructions before entering the temple.

[previous page] Light through trellis at Humanyn's Tomb
[opposite] Dusty streets of Old Delhi

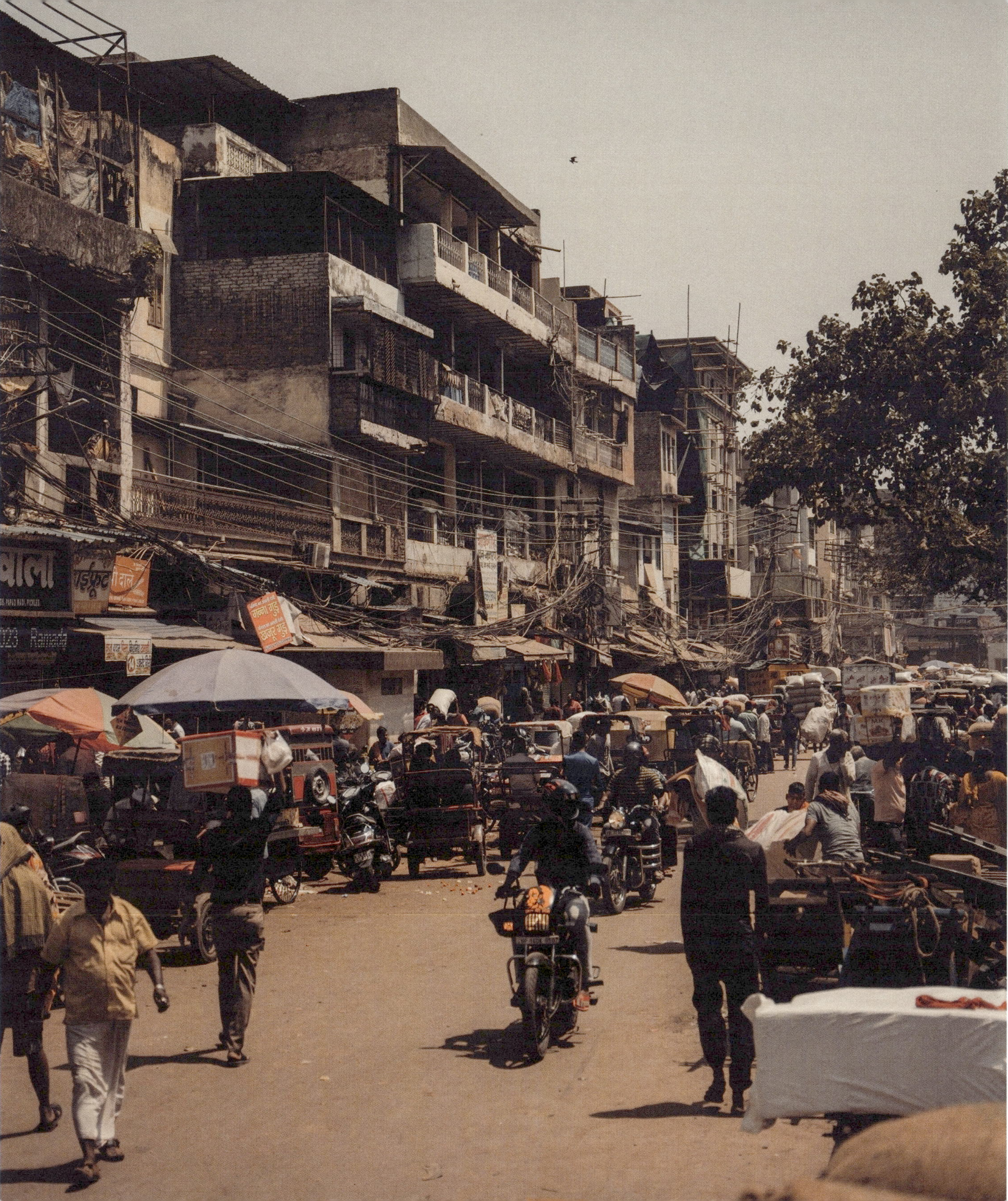

Ramada
खजूर गुड़

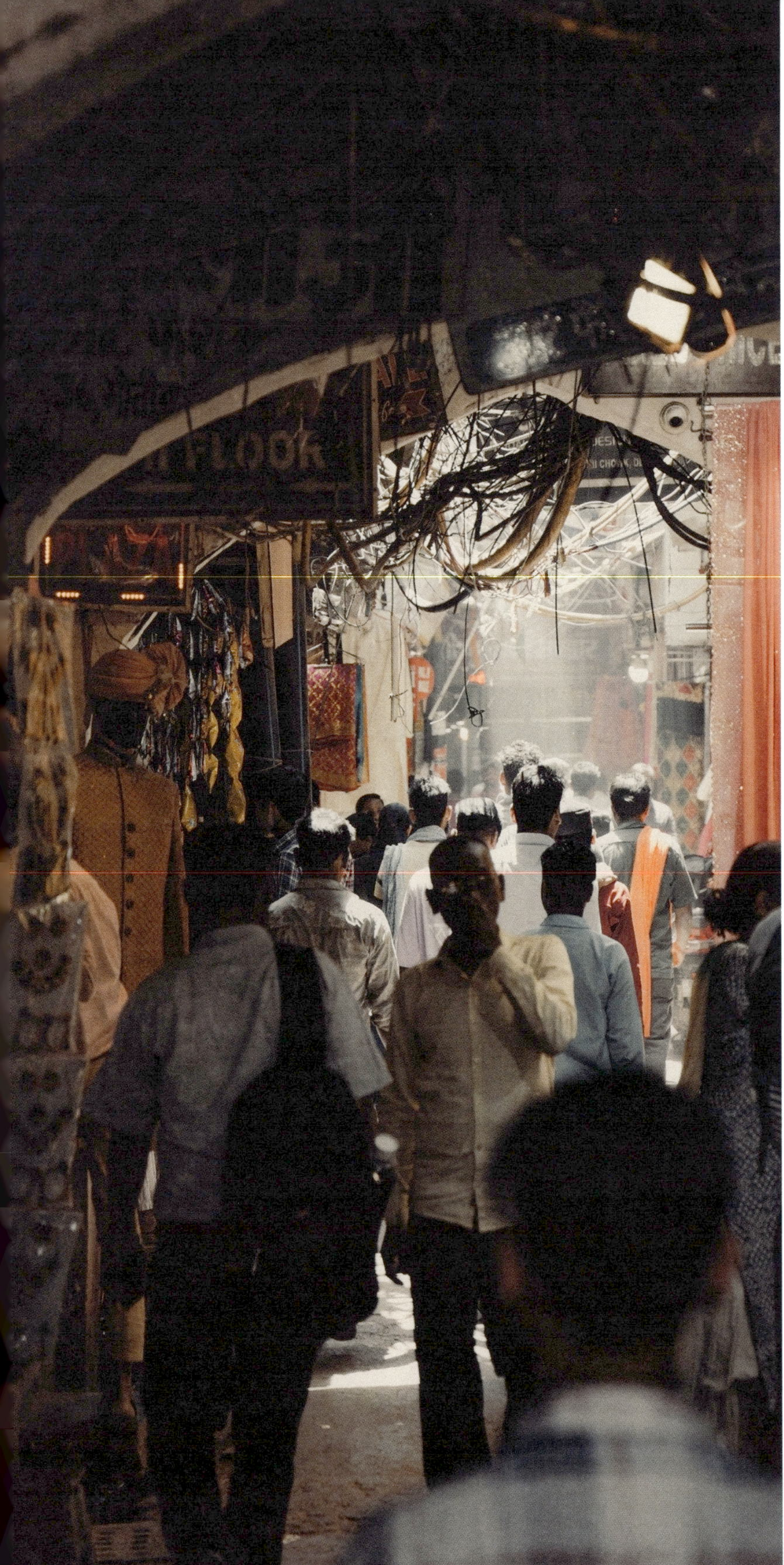

I walk through a tapestry of colours, encountering symbols, sculptures, and paintings at every turn. The Hindu goddess Durga and the elephant-headed god Ganesha are among the deities portrayed in the temple. At the altar, I present a tray of sweets, as instructed. The priest keeps some of the offering at the altar and returns the rest, pouring water into my cupped hands. This act of *achamana* symbolizes purification and cleansing of the mind and senses. With orange paint, known as tilaka, dotting my forehead, I feel accepted and welcomed. Observing individuals praying and moving from deity to deity, I witness a very personal and independent nature to their worship. People come and go, some praying for support, others exuding joy. It's a beautiful reminder that the path to spiritual fulfillment is deeply personal, and each individual finds their own unique connection with something greater than themselves. Leaving the temple, I offer the remaining sweets to a homeless man, who receives them with gratitude.

The presence and coexistence of religious activities is evident to me. We wander through holy sites of different faiths and are welcomed and accepted. India is home to a variety of spiritual practices. The reverence for faith and religion in India serves as an ever-present reminder of its universal role in its peoples' lives.

Continuing our journey, we stroll down busy streets lined with shops showcasing intricate wedding gowns, gold jewellery, and textiles. The brightly decorated windows attract shoppers, and the never-ending crowd pushes us forward. Eventually, we reach a large open space on the sidewalk, where piles of grain lie as a community kitchen prepares free meals for the less fortunate. Volunteers hustle about, demonstrating care and generosity. Regardless of status, religion, or background, all are welcome to partake in the nourishment provided.

After some bargaining with a driver, we grab a tuk-tuk to our next destination, a massive mausoleum called Humayun's Tomb, nestled into sprawling gardens on all sides. This impressive structure, the final resting place of the Mughal

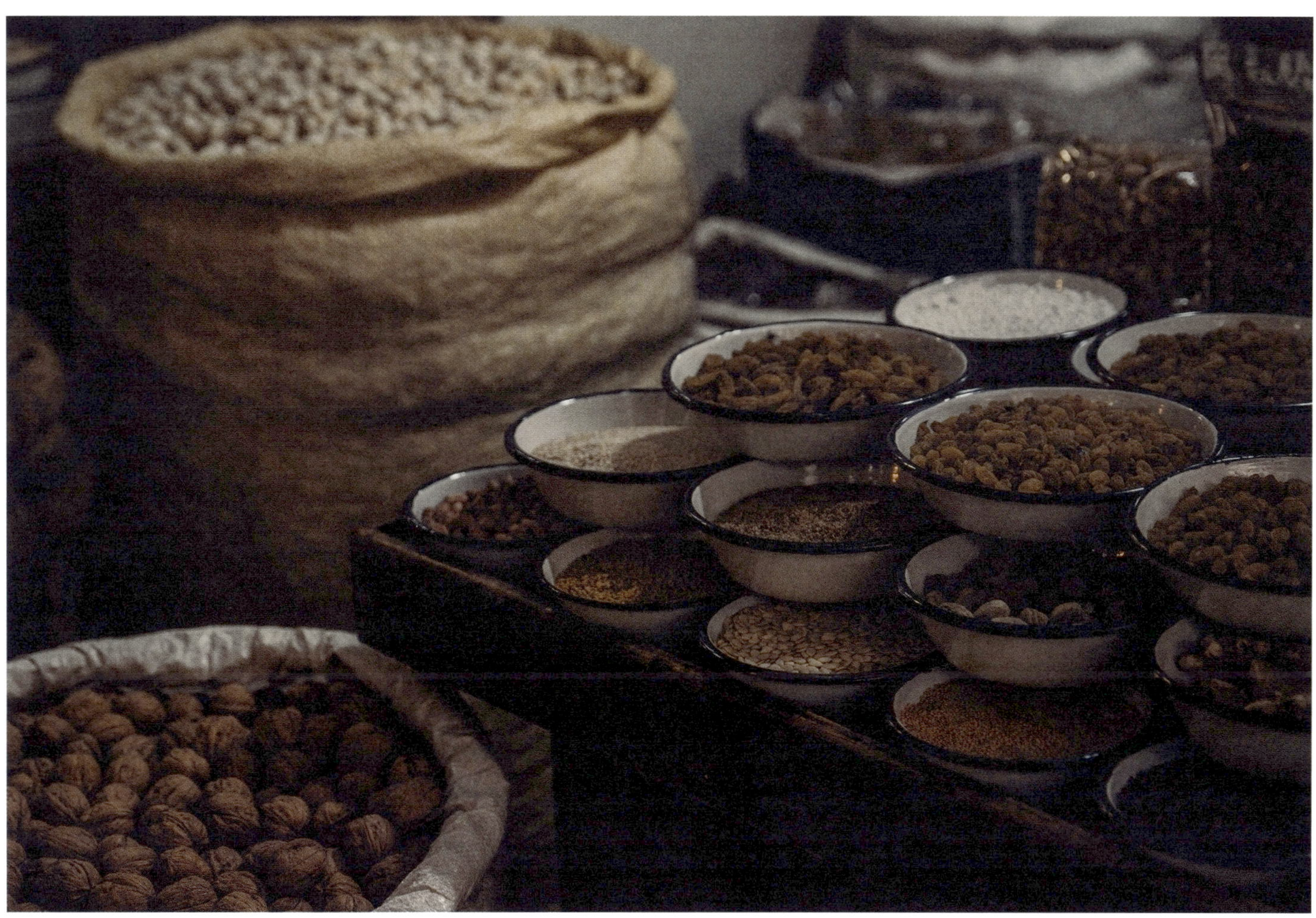

emperor, Humayun, showcases the rich architectural heritage of its time and serves as a peaceful oasis in the heart of Delhi.

I walk through the main gates toward the domed structure. The setting sun reflects off its red sandstone facade. Intricate white designs adorn the stone, leading me to the entrance of the tomb. Inside, delicate marble lattice screens allow rays of sunlight to dance on the cool stone floors. I find calm in the quiet and move to the north side of the terrace, leaning against the railing to take in the scene. Birds sing and dart across the sky as the sun dips below the horizon, casting a warm glow upon the tomb. In that moment, surrounded by the beauty of nature, I find relief from the day's excitement. The blue sky above turns yellow as the crimson orange creeps over the horizon. I watch in reflective silence as the daylight fades. Reluctantly, I rise from my perch, ready to embark on the journey back. I stroll through the parks and yards of the tomb as the city sounds gradually grow with each step.

I emerge from the site to an intersection and expressway and find our vehicle ready to pick us up. The seemingly perfect timing among the chaotic traffic amazes me after hours of wandering. Fatigued yet invigorated, we begin the voyage back to our hotel, weaving through the busy streets.

[opposite] Bustling alleys of central Delhi
[above] Spices, spices, and more spices

A DAY OF DISCOVERY

A warm fog rises and lingers between the trees. The sun's first rays creep through the leaves and warm the faces of the yogis doing their morning practice in the park. I wander through Lodi Gardens, passing group after group of people stretching, meditating, laughing, working out, and communing. Groups of people dot the lawns, walkers pace by, and chatters converse through their morning strolls. This is a quiet haven of the city, a sacred nature sanctuary and a refuge for peace and mindfulness. Witnessing the value placed on these practices, I immerse myself in the peaceful ambiance, rejuvenated and ready for the day ahead.

Leaving the garden, I meet my guide, and we head toward our ultimate destination. Driving through the ever-expanding city, we observe the changing landscape, from historical monuments to towering apartment buildings. Finally, we arrive at a small school dedicated to underprivileged children living in poverty-stricken conditions. Here, they not only receive a basic education but also learn mindfulness practices to help navigate the challenges of life. Singing, dancing, meditating, and practising yoga are integrated into their curriculum alongside traditional subjects. It is called the "School of Happiness," and we are their honoured guests for the day.

Greeted with warmth and respect, we are welcomed into the school by Munesh, a spiritual teacher, friend, and advocate for the children. Scarves are draped around our necks as we bow, allowing the students to place flower necklaces over our heads. The children are clad in matching blue jumpsuits; their innocent faces beam with curiosity and joy. Led inside the modest building, we receive an orange tika on our foreheads, a humble gesture accompanied by a few grains of rice pressed into the paint. We are then guided to our seats and the assembly commences with the announcement of our names. The children respond in unison, their coordinated roar welcoming us with their school's mantra. We are treated to a series of traditional songs, dances, and poetry recitals, eventually joining in the cheerful dance party. Fully engaged and present, we experience the power of mindfulness and awareness. The children remind me of the children I know back home, radiating happiness and innocence and the universality of youth.

The next task is to provide food for the children, a humbling and eye-opening experience. Serving those children makes me acutely aware of the triviality of my own problems and challenges. Our host masterfully intertwines joy and reality in our experience, revealing the children's gratitude and appreciation in the face of seemingly insurmountable obstacles. The ability to find positivity and express gratitude in the direst of circumstances is a testament to their resilience. I cannot recall another moment where I have been so simultaneously full of joy and sorrow. It is a duality of emotion that is challenging to grasp.

After the school day concludes, we walk to Munesh's home to engage in meaningful conversation with him and his family. As we chat and share food, I can't help but feel a deep sense of connection and kinship. Indian culture emphasizes spirituality and the recognition of the divine presence in all beings, and this is palpable in every interaction. The concept of "Karma" and the pursuit of selfless actions and hospitality are deeply ingrained in their way of life. As Munesh enlightens me about the perspectives I have been experiencing in my time in India, I feel a profound shift in my understanding and awareness of Indian culture. Hours pass as we share stories and philosophy in his home.

Seeing curiosity sparked in me, Munesh leaves me with a statement to ponder: "The streets of Delhi appear chaotic, but to those who call it home, there is order within."

In the weeks that follow, I delve into the depths of this statement. It becomes clear that many assumptions about India's ancient traditions have been distorted or selectively filtered through our Western lens. Yoga, for instance, is more than mere exercise; it encompasses a profound spiritual journey of self-discovery, connection, and balance. Mindfulness is woven into the fabric of India's spiritual traditions, enabling individuals to find harmony and inner peace amidst the bustling chaos of everyday life.

Thus, while the streets of Delhi may appear chaotic to outsiders, those who call it home discover their own order within . . . a reflection of their own being. In the West, we have a seemingly orderly society but bear the burden of enormous mental health challenges and struggle with chaos in our minds.

The recognition that inner peace can be discovered amid turmoil serves as a potent reminder that true harmony originates from within. It is through the trials and tribulations of our existence that the profound beauty and serenity of our reality can be unveiled. It may be that the chaos itself enables us to fully appreciate tranquility and find comfort in calm.

Humanyun's Tomb at sundown

A HEALTHY MIND AND SPIRIT

By applying these takeaways we can cultivate a sense of balance, inner peace, and interconnectedness with ourselves and those around us. Whenever possible, try to embrace mindfulness, gratitude, respect, generosity, and personal growth. You may find your perspective expands and your experiences are enriched.

MIND YOUR WELL-BEING: Stress, anxiety, and depression have all been reduced through regular mindfulness practices. By addressing your mental health challenges, you can promote emotional resilience and foster a more positive outlook in daily life.

KNOW THYSELF: Introspection and self-reflection allow you to better know yourself. It gives you insights into triggers, emotional patterns, and barriers that keep you from reaching your full potential. Dive deep into your thoughts and see what you discover. Perform acts of service, volunteer, or support causes that resonate with you. Helping others is an easy way to help gain a perspective about how lucky you are.

FIND FOCUS: In a world that demands your attention, you need to learn how to focus your mind and stay on task. Regular meditation and mindfulness practices hone your skills and allow you to better control your attention. Be mindful of the sights, sounds, smells, tastes, and feelings you experience.

BE HUMAN: Mindfulness practices draw you into the present moment. This reduces your stress, improves perspective, and creates an environment where you can shut down ruminating thoughts and break harmful patterns. Seek knowledge and understand the diversity of different beliefs. Engage in respectful conversation and learn about how others achieve mindfulness through culture and tradition.

BE EMOTIONALLY AGILE: Your emotions can change after a single interaction, but practising mindfulness allows you to better navigate your emotions. Spirituality creates a better sense of curiosity and compassion for others and allows you to take things less personally while appreciating other perspectives with patience.

GROW RESILIENCE: By improving your sense of connection, purpose, and adaptability through mindfulness and spirituality, you can weather the storms of life and better recover from stressful situations.

OUR MINDFUL MENTORS

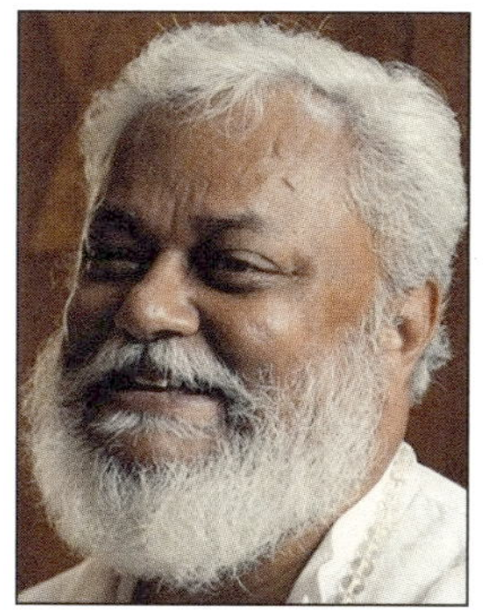

MUNESH: As a spiritual leader and dedicated community volunteer, through his organization, The School of Happiness, Munesh offers invaluable support to underprivileged youth, helping them overcome the challenges they face in their daily lives while balancing their education. His message revolves around acceptance, finding harmony, purpose, and the transformative power of acts of service. His ability to inspire and mentor others has gained him international recognition for his insightful teachings and unique perspectives on mindfulness. Munesh's work has touched the lives of many, leaving a lasting impact on those fortunate enough to learn from him.

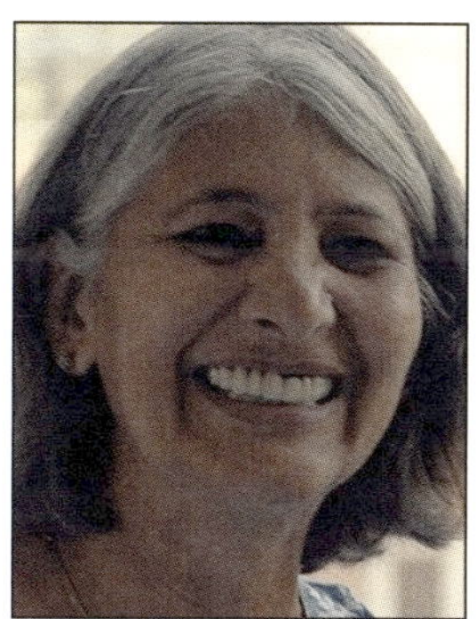

HASHMITA: I was fortunate enough to meet Hashmita on my travels in Delhi. Embodying dedication and wisdom, she is a lifelong student of the human experience and a practitioner of Dharma. Her profound understanding of Karma and its significance in Indian culture enriched our journey, offering invaluable insights as we explored the country. Her grace and eloquence in sharing her knowledge left a deep impression on us, deepening our understanding of the universal importance of acts of service, kindness, and generosity. Through her teachings, we realized that these values transcend religious boundaries and should be treasured by all, regardless of one's background, ethnicity, or spiritual beliefs.

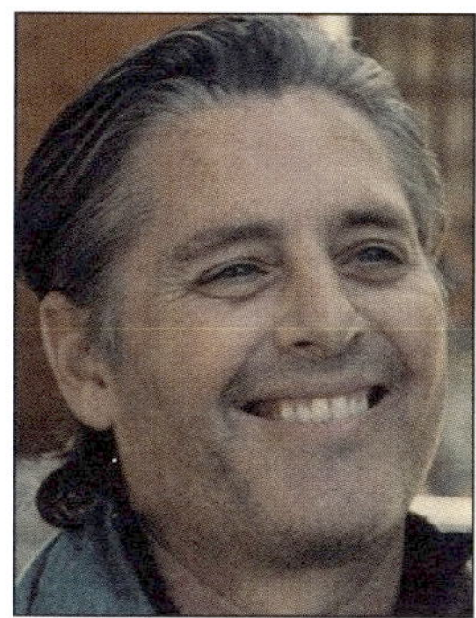

JESSE STIRLING: Jesse is a close friend whose love for India inspired my visit. He is a Western interpreter of mindfulness practices in India, a kindred spirit in his love of the world and its people. His deep connection to the country spans generations, inspired by his family's three-generation pilgrimages to Northern India. Jesse's unique ability to integrate the teachings of spirituality into his everyday life back home in Canada serves as a creative demonstration of the universality of these practices. His insights and experiences have been shared in a captivating TED Talk on meditation entitled, "Two lungs, two eyelids, two minutes," which inspires others to embrace mindfulness and seamlessly incorporate it into their own lives.

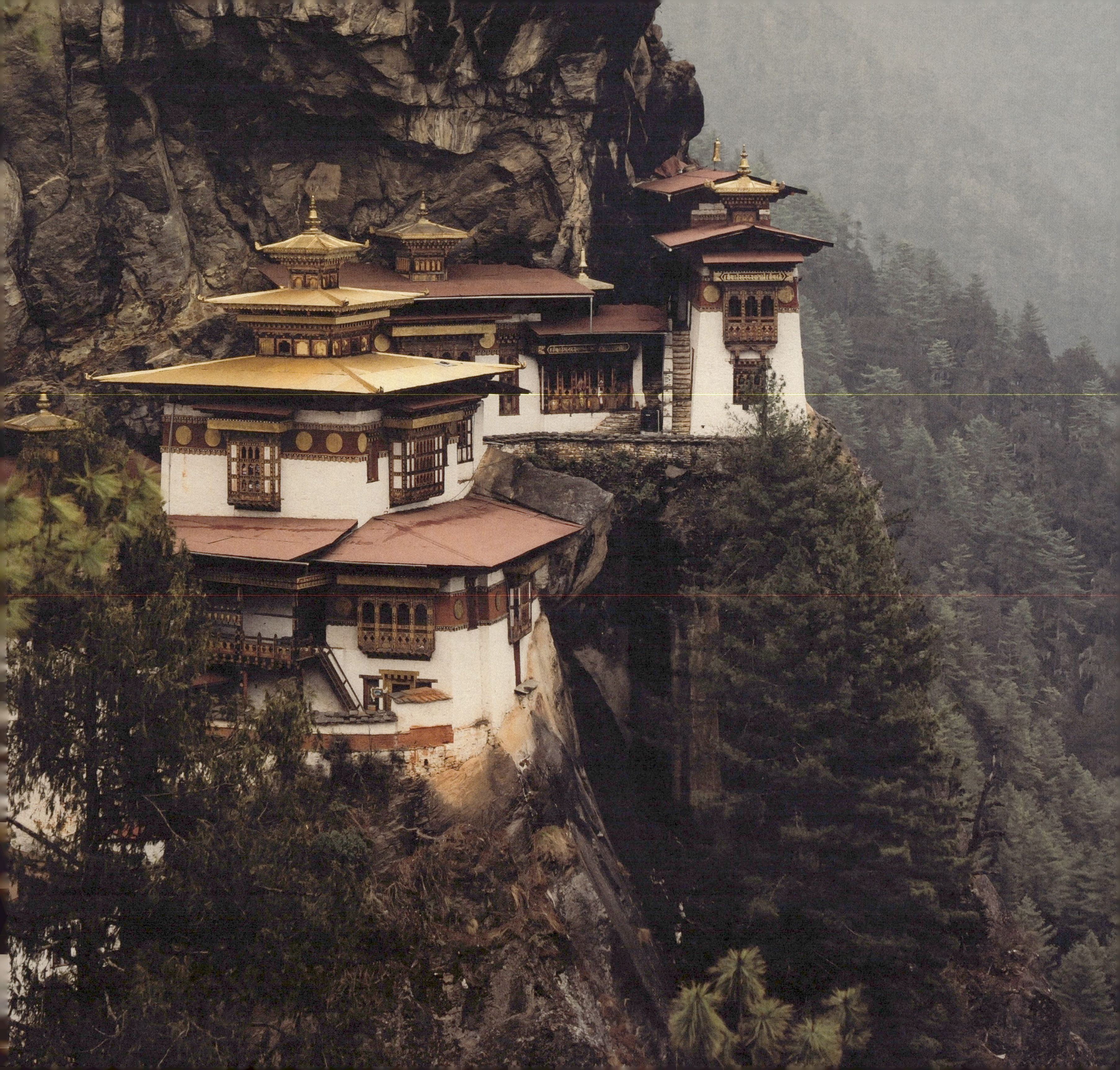

4

THE PURSUIT OF HAPPINESS

Among the hurry and stress of the modern world, the hidden kingdom of Bhutan offers a way of life that encourages its people—officially—to seek happiness and balance. Just as Bhutan's landscapes provide a refuge for nurturing well-being, its society cherishes happiness as a precious resource within its community.

FINDING HAPPINESS

Gazing out of the airplane window, my eyes fix on the magnificent peaks of the Himalayas of Bhutan. I can't help but reflect on the significance of this journey. The valley below, where the capital city of Thimphu is nestled, seems like a magical place that exists only in legends.

Descending into this otherworldly realm takes expertise that only eight pilots in the world possess. Our aviators skillfully maneuver our plane through the treacherous cliffs. The calming Bhutanese music playing in the cabin can't quell the flickers of anxiety in my mind. Never before have I started a flight descent in which high-altitude clouds are replaced by rock faces and trees. They flash by my window, and my mind struggles to fathom the magnitude of these mountains. Yet, despite my apprehension, I know the rewards awaiting me in the happiest kingdom on Earth—a place that has eluded so many, both figuratively and literally—will make it all worthwhile.

This pilgrimage to Bhutan is not purely one of curiosity; it is deeply personal for me.

To truly appreciate the significance of this journey, I must first reflect on my father and a promise that I made to him. He was a remarkable man—a modern-day Indiana Jones, alternating between his roles as a highly educated geological consultant and prospector, and a loving family man. I recall the story of his meeting my mother after he moved from Colorado to New Brunswick. He stood out in sleepy Fredericton with his stetson cowboy hat, Hudson Bay jacket, and leather mukluks. He met my mother, a collegiate diver and straight-A student, through mutual friends. They were an unconventional couple, but their connection was instantaneous, and they fell in love at first sight. One might think it was his adventurous spirit she loved, but she will say it was his gentle demeanor and beaming kindness.

He was the most supportive father a son could ask for. He guided me in life with a spark of encouragement that always accompanied my ideas and sometimes held back practical advice to preserve my enthusiasm. He never ceased to amaze me, constantly pivoting between working on home projects,

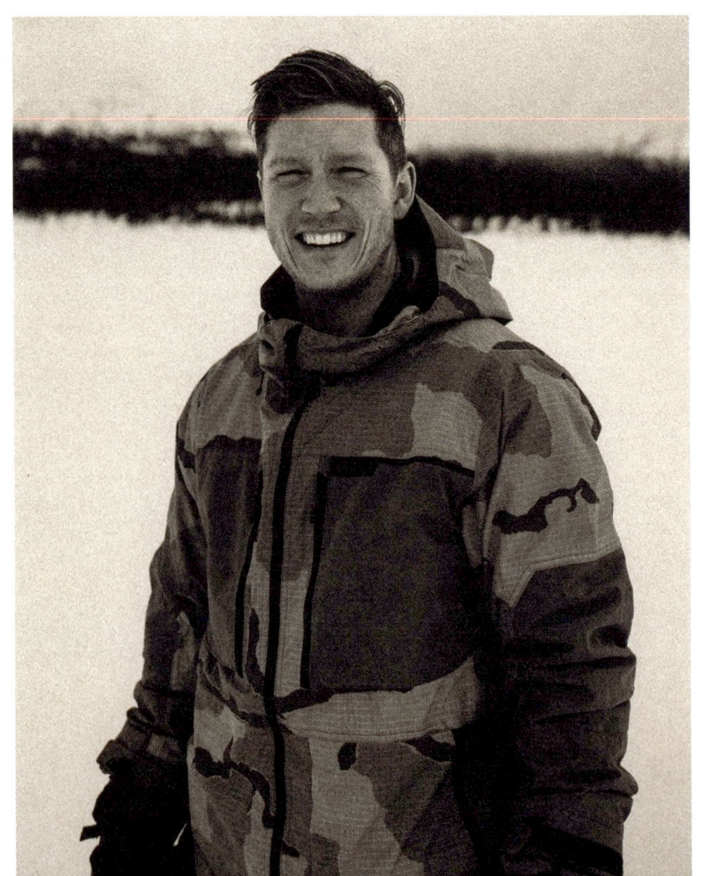

drawing geological maps by hand that belonged in museums, or finding ways to recycle and repurpose materials—years ahead of his time with his environmental consciousness. Unlike my mother, whose entrepreneurial spirit thrived in a formal setting, he undertook consulting projects, departing to Albania for two months, or setting up a prospecting camp in King Bay, in Northern Ontario, when winter broke. I recall the excitement when he developed film after trips, a nostalgic reminder of my pre-digital childhood. I spent a great deal of time in his company. He was not only my father but also my best friend—a confidant with whom I shared every piece of news.

Then suddenly, everything changed. It was during my early thirties when my father's health began to decline. He began to slow down, plagued by persistent stomach pain that refused to relent. The initial diagnosis of bladder cancer filled our hearts with fear, yet the prospects of recovery provided a glimmer of hope. However, our hopes were swiftly shattered when we discovered that pancreatic cancer had stealthily taken hold. In the face of this cruel reality, he fought valiantly, battling for eight arduous months. Throughout it all, he shielded me from the full extent of his suffering.

Not long before he passed, I took a trip home to visit him. At this time, he could still engage with me and spend quality time together. We sat quietly outside in the sun, overlooking the backyard he had so carefully cultivated for decades. I knew my flight was leaving in an hour, but I wanted to make the moment last. My hands were fidgeting, unsure about what to do, knowing that this would likely be one of the last times I would be in his company.

His eyes teared up, and he grasped my nervous hands with intention. I remember looking down at his fingers as they gripped me tight, his hands strong and weathered even in his fragile state. It brought me out of my thoughts and into the present moment that I had been avoiding. Staring deeply into my eyes, he said, "You have to promise me something when I'm gone." The permanence of his words pierced my heart. "Of course, whatever you want. What is it?" I stammered.

"I want you to find happiness."

He squeezed my hand and smiled in an unbelievable show of appreciation that any moment holds the opportunity for beauty, even one as sad as a goodbye.

That was the last face-to-face conversation I had with my father.

His condition quickly deteriorated in the weeks that followed until that fateful day when my mother's call urged me to rush back to New Brunswick. I arrived in Fredericton that afternoon, only to witness his body failing, his strength ebbing away. My presence offered him the opportunity to say goodbye and the permission to move on to his next adventure. In those final moments, as his life slipped away, he looked at me and I remembered his simple yet resolute request.

At first, the wish seemed puzzling. After all, I believed I was content in life—I had a fulfilling job and was in a long-term relationship, I was close to finishing my PhD, and by societal standards, I was successful. Yet, his passing left an enormous void in my life, and when I turned to those outside of my family that I considered closest, I found I was very much alone.

The ensuing years became a period of introspection, where my understanding of my relationship with others and the world, the importance of life's balance, and my very definition of success underwent a radical transformation. I separated from my romantic partner shortly after returning to Newfoundland from the funeral, and within twelve months, my relationship with my long-time business partner and friend had soured, and I bought him out. It was then that I started to surround myself with a truly supportive community.

I began to comprehend that my father's request had not been made lightly; it was a culmination of years of withheld advice, masterfully surfacing in a moment timed to ensure that I listened when it mattered most.

[page 52] The Tiger's Nest Temple
[opposite] Labrador in black and white

THE KINGDOM OF HAPPINESS

A decade has passed since I made that promise, and my thoughts snap back to the present moment as our plane lands in Bhutan. Exiting the aircraft, a refreshing breeze from the mountains envelops me. I collect my bags and am greeted warmly by our guide, whose name, surprisingly, is Karma. Clad in traditional Bhutanese attire enhanced with a modern grey-patterned fabric, his hair is neatly trimmed and polarized sunglasses swing from a string around his neck; he exudes an air of readiness that stems from his military background.

Karma exemplifies his name, a concept that will resonate during our week together. I don't yet know how much insight I will gain about the land and its people from our interactions with him. His natural ability to forge connections, spread joy, and share lighthearted humour consistently rejuvenates our spirits, countering the fatigue of the journey.

We have come to Bhutan because it stands alone as a country that measures its progress, in part, with a unique system: Gross National Happiness (GNH). Bhutan's devotion to balanced development, cultural preservation, and social unity offers a potent reminder that authentic prosperity stems from intertwining material growth with the richness of human experience. In short, it is officially devoted to advancing happiness.

Our first stop provides insight into how Bhutanese individuals spend their weekends. We navigate winding mountain roads from the airport to Thimphu—a city that seems suspended in time, where architectural traditions thrive. Every corner reveals grand edifices adorned with intricate woodwork, ornate paintings, and traditional roofs, their white facades dominating the scenery. Pristine streets reflect the city's dedication to cleanliness, while the air itself carries an extraordinary purity, a testament to Bhutan's status as the world's sole carbon-neutral nation. Wending our way through the city's streets, we reach an archery field, an arena where Bhutanese life unfolds.

This archery ground serves as a communal hub where men engage in good-natured competition. Their partners cheer them on, offering support and beverages (some stronger than others) as archers expertly launch arrows, hitting astonishing distances of 200 metres with their traditional bows. Playfully, the opposing team at the target teases and jokes as their rivals shoot skyward, often only narrowly missing their mark. Stories of participants deflecting arrows with their clothing are commonplace, as an arrow wound apparently stings less than defeat.

Less than an hour has passed since our arrival, and I am staring across the archery field awestruck at where I find myself. Dozens of archers dot the field, their colourful clothing so different and unique, and I begin to realize that this place will forever etch itself into my memory.

In this atmosphere of recreation, archers welcome us, showcasing their skills and playfully taunting one another for errant shots. Karma, himself an archer, weaves us into the festivities. He directs us to film as he engages in lively conversations with friends and provides animated commentary on the competition. After somehow striking the tiny target, the archers burst into a jubilant dance called the Langtsho. This dance embodies the camaraderie shared by participants and observers alike. Pausing the game, they synchronize their movements. Harmonious singing echoes across the archery grounds.

Back and forth they move and sing in their traditional garb, drawing attention to the success of their competitor in a strangely respectful celebration of the other team's accomplishment. It reminds me of an NFL touchdown dance—only one performed by the team that was just scored upon. My Western sports' mind argues with itself over this tradition, but the win-at-all-costs spirit of competition is extinguished by a layer of adversarial admiration and respect. As the dance crescendos, archers raise their hands in unison, bows and arrows aligned, and with a triumphant "Waho, Waho, Waho," they conclude their celebration.

Witnessing this display of sportsmanship offers a glimpse into the Bhutanese people's capacity to cherish even the smallest victories, fostering community bonds and embracing life's joyful moments. Throughout, I see Karma, an energetic participant, celebrate alongside the archers, inviting me to join in the final chorus of resonating "Wahos!"

Next, we wander to a lively traditional market. Stalls overflow with a rainbow of colourful vegetables and local produce. One aisle brims with fiery peppers, another with farm-fresh vegetables, while yet another showcases dried fish and other unfamiliar ingredients. Among the conversations and

[above] Prayer flags on mountain trail

crowds of shoppers, tiny children trail me with interest. As I meander through the vibrant market, a sense of carefree spirit envelops me, immersing me in the rhythm of Bhutanese life. Every sight, sound, and aroma acts to demonstrate how here, contentment and simplicity reign.

Amidst this bustling marketplace, we gain an intimate view of local customs. Karma introduces us to a friendly vendor who generously treats me to freshly made dumplings. Opening a heated container, she heaps the delicate delights onto small paper plates. After savouring one, I praise her culinary skills with respectful bows and grateful expressions, conveying my appreciation more effectively than our attempts at the Bhutanese language can. She refuses payment, instead eager to share her traditional delicacies. This modest moment is a departure from the typical tourist experience, where hospitality typically comes with inflated fees that too often overshadow a delicious moment.

Leaving the market behind, we venture into a tranquil corner where children play happily with tree blossoms, their laughter bounding through the air. School having concluded for the day, the young girls toss the pink petals skyward, then twirl in the falling flowers with glee. They giggle and grin as their beautiful confetti falls to the stones, making me smile. After they have collected all the petals within their reach, I volunteer to reach higher blossoms, presenting them with another handful of smiles. Eagerly they signal for more, and I continue to pick the flowers until their hands overflow. With a Bhutanese count to three, they release the petals. A chorus of cheers follows. There's a shared anticipation and a sense of wonder as we engage in the children's game. Their pride in their performance brings us joy.

Eventually, we bow and wave, and we continue on toward the shouts and cheers we hear around the corner. Approaching the town square, we see a group of boys engage in an animated soccer match. Seeing our cameras, they warmly invite me to join, and I eagerly become part of their game.

"Where are you from?" one asks, and I say, "Canada." Another boy, fluent in English, shares a wealth of facts about my country with his friend. Before he finishes explaining Canada's status as the second largest country in the world, the ball is back in play, and the game continues. The young men shout, slide and kick, increasing the game's intensity with an adult present to show off for. Our team presses forward and kicks the ball between the two stone goal posts . . . Gooooaaaaalllllll!

Our collective celebration is marked by high-fives and laughter from both sides. I retire and let them continue unimpeded by their geriatric teammate.

During these precious moments—whether exploring the bustling market, observing children's delight in blossoms, engaging in soccer, or even during the archery competition—I feel an intense connection and sense of belonging. Bhutan's people, with their open hearts and open minds, bridge gaps effortlessly, making me feel not only welcome but also valued as a guest in their community. This seems to be inherent to them as a people, and I wonder how this can be fostered so universally in their community.

These experiences illuminate the transformative power of genuine human connections and the remarkable ease with which the Bhutanese people embrace others, irrespective of the divides that often plague East-West connections. It serves as a poignant reminder that true happiness resides in life's simple pleasures, the warmth of human connections, and the embrace of the present moment.

As night falls and I prepare for bed, I reflect on the day. From childhood, my father had urged me to mine diamonds in life—a reference not only to his career as a geologist but also to a philosophy ingrained in my upbringing. "Diamonds," he'd say, "are small yet valuable, much like these moments. You don't need many to experience richness in life."

So, I tuck the precious moments of the day into my memory and my heart, thanking my father for his wisdom before drifting into a peaceful sleep.

[opposite] Royal Botanical Garden Serbithang

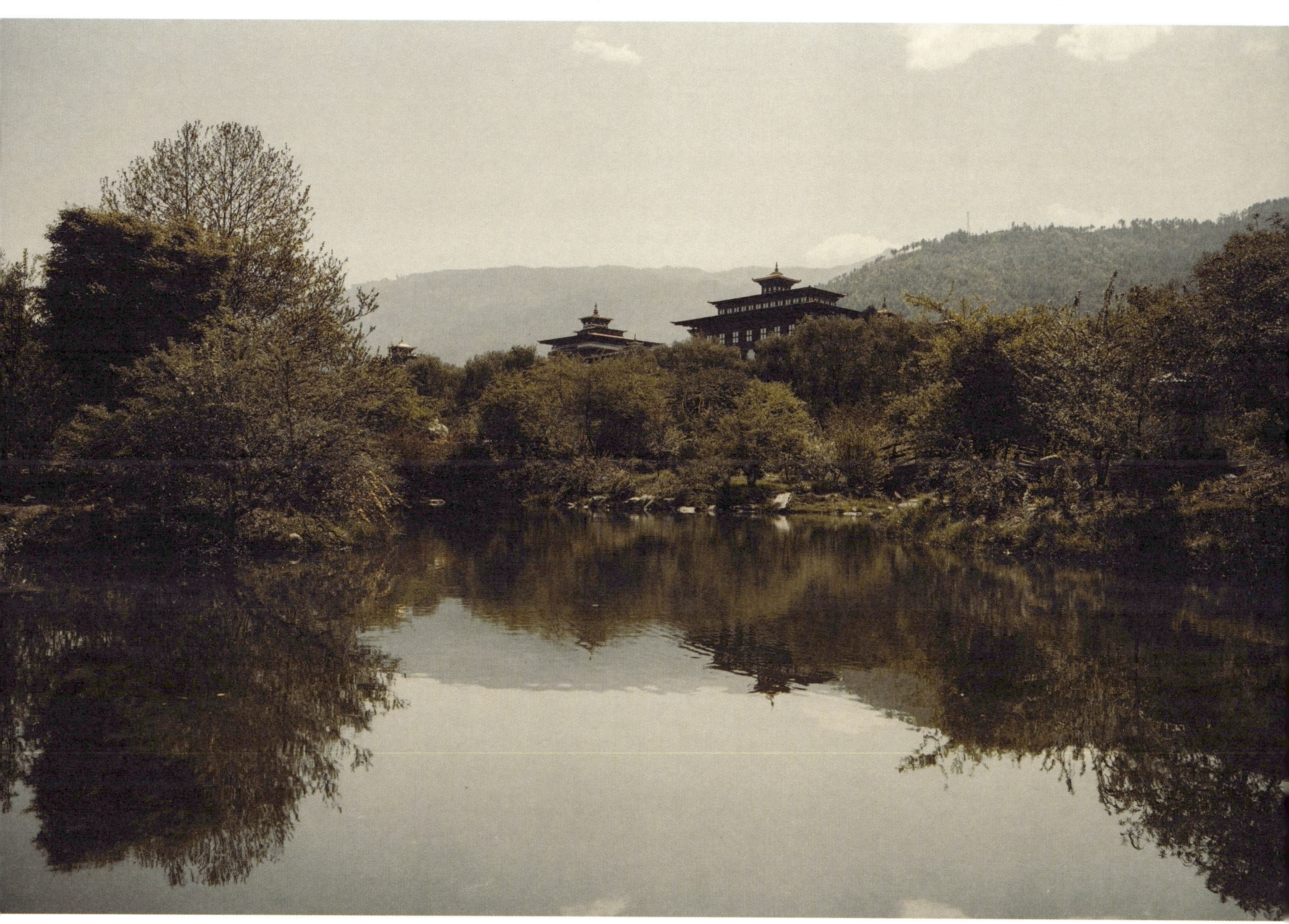

GOOD KARMA

Throughout the journey, my guide Karma emerges as a focal point. Karma is no stranger to leading expeditions for both adventure enthusiasts and storytellers alike. He recently guided Will Smith during his time in Bhutan and boasts a portfolio of previous documentaries he has been a part of. With a versatile skill set that spans cultural tours, fishing excursions, and hiking and climbing adventures, he embodies a wealth of knowledge. As he advanced in his career, he assumed a leadership role within his organization only to swiftly realize that the trappings of office work didn't align with his outgoing nature. This realization propelled him back into the field, where his true passion resides. That passion intertwines his journey with mine.

Karma's expertise proves invaluable as he helps organize my destinations, ensuring an authentic immersion into Bhutanese culture. One particularly memorable stop leads me to the awe-inspiring Buddha Dordenma statue, which commands a panoramic view over Thimphu, the capital city. It is here that Karma shares the legend of Buddha. Patiently guiding me through the scene, he engages in on-camera discussions, directing our team to capture respectful shots while advising on optimal angles, lighting, and timing.

As we venture into the rustic landscapes of Punakha, Karma's importance on our trip becomes even more apparent. Recognizing the constraints imposed by ongoing elections, which limit traditional performances, Karma thoughtfully organizes a private cultural exhibition for us. This gesture ensures that I can still partake in the local celebrations specific to Bhutan's cultural history, known as a Tshechu festival. Karma borrows a flute to play a song while we wait for the performance to begin. Expecting a lively tune, I am surprised as a quiet

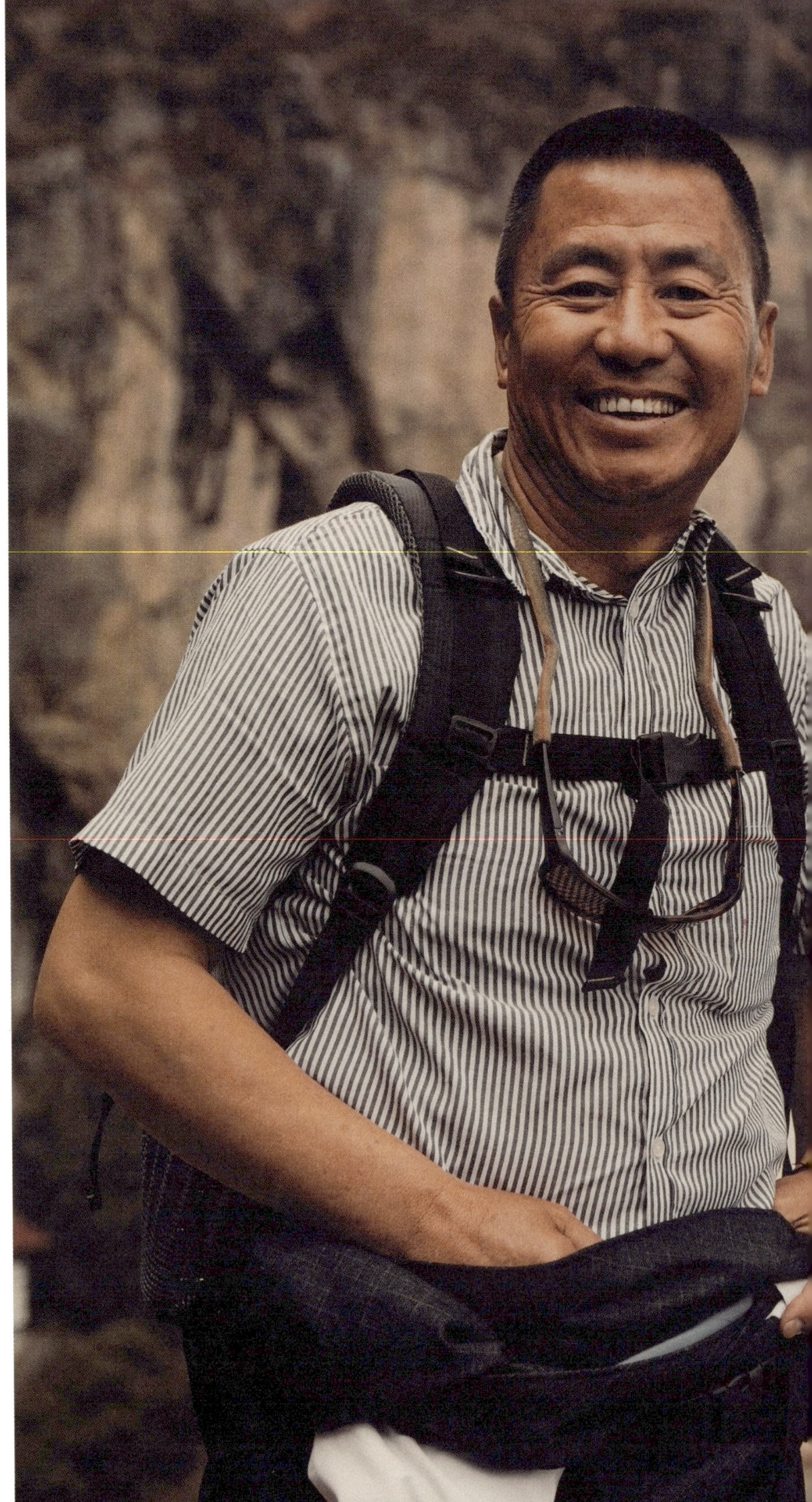

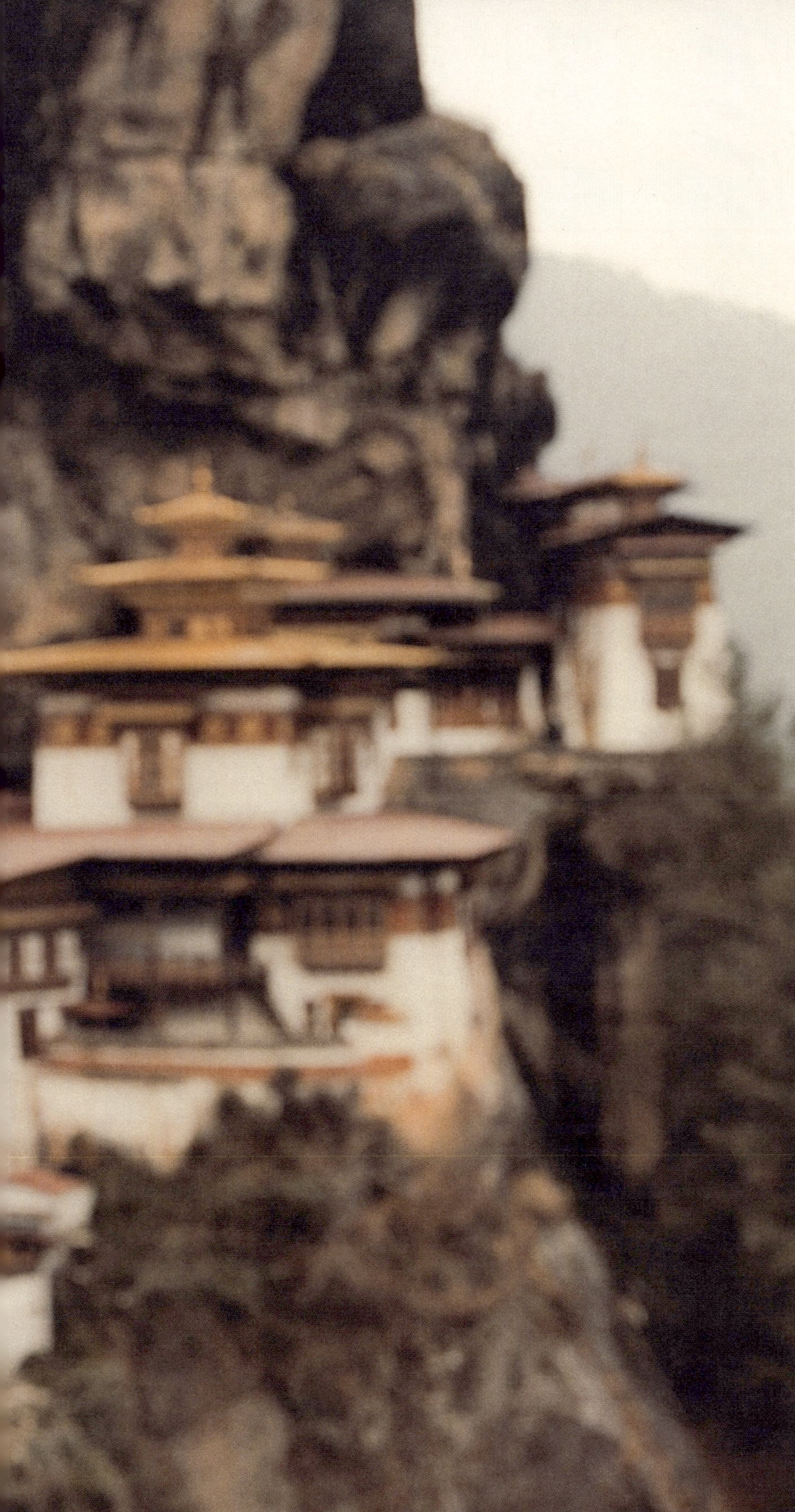

melody floats through the room. I feel myself breathe out the day's stress as the music acts to settle the room and creates a crispness of consciousness. It seems intentional to bring our attention to the spectacle we're about to witness and I am grateful for the reminder.

We later visited a rural school where I had the opportunity to discuss teaching philosophy with Principal Youten Jamtsho, and it was Karma's connections that opened the door to my understanding.

Beyond his role as a guide, Karma maintains a sense of equilibrium and thoughtfulness that leaves an indelible mark. During my visit to a rural farmhouse, arranged through a Bhutanese education colleague of mine, Karma guides me with attentiveness through the intricacies of the local customs. He ensures I navigate the cultural nuances with respect, all the while safeguarding my well-being by alerting me to potentially unsafe water sources without offending our gracious hosts. At that farmhouse, Karma orchestrates an archery tournament, affording me the opportunity to partake in this traditional Bhutanese sport. Amid our celebrations of a successful shot, a small group of us unite in the Langtsho dance—a moment encapsulating the bond formed, with Karma steering our journey.

Karma isn't just a resourceful guide—he also acts with great kindness during times of need. When Braeden contracts gastroenteritis from contaminated water, Karma springs into action. He swiftly coordinates with a doctor, and we pick up the physician from the hospital, who accompanies us to our mountaintop hotel—an establishment that boasts breathtaking views but is hardly a practical setting for medical treatment.

Throughout this voyage, it feels as if destiny has graced us with the remarkable fortune of having Karma as our guide. His very name echoes the harmonious energy shared by the Bhutanese people. He gives me a glimpse into the way of life and the values the community holds dear: kindness, happiness, and hospitality.

Karma Tschering—a guide and friend

THE PATH TO HAPPINESS

As my visit to Bhutan nears its end, my final destination awaits me in Paro–Taktsang, also known as the Tiger's Nest, the revered birthplace of Buddhism in Bhutan. To reach this sacred site, we embark on a horseback journey, slowly ascending to 3300 metres. The rhythmic and steady steps of our durable horses are an experience I'll remember. Ironically, the horses favour walking on the barely five-centimetre-wide trail that borders a steep drop of over a thousand metres, their wide torsos hiding their feet so that looking off the edge provides a terrifying perception of flying. I nickname my horse Pegasus for this illusion.

Several times the butterflies in my stomach and common sense nearly win the battle and I catch myself pushing up on the saddle to dismount and walk my horse up the mountain. But each time my shoulders relax and I fall back into the leather seat, a reluctant victory over fear. Side to side, step after step the horses climb. As we approach 2500 metres above sea level, I recall a hiking experience in the Andes a decade earlier and the breathlessness of altitude, and I stay firmly anchored in the saddle. My lungs thank me for the reprieve.

My senses heighten with anticipation as I near the drop-off point two-thirds of the way up the mountain. From there, the path transforms into a trail we have to conquer on foot, ascending the final 800 metres.

The high-altitude hike pushes me to my limits as I trudge toward the summit. Prayer flags adorn the trail, gently swaying in the mountain breeze, imbuing the surroundings with a sense of spiritual tranquility. As we press forward, we encounter fellow travellers making their way back down, their faces reflecting the awe-inspiring experience they've just had. Behind me is Karma, strolling with his hands held behind his back, his melodious whistling providing a soothing ambiance to my ascent.

The night before, in a moment of contemplation, a realization had stirred in me, prompting me to write a letter to my father—a message of gratitude to be left at this symbolic location. In that note, I express my appreciation for his request that I find happiness. As I contemplate the things that I am truly grateful for, I discover that they are the intangible treasures of life—my sense of peace and serenity, the ability to embark on transformative journeys, the bonds with friends, family, and community. The love I've found for my wife, Leanne. These are the things that were absent in the past. I recognize the lasting impact of my father's mentorship, even long after his physical presence has departed.

Travelling to Bhutan was not a quest to find happiness but a catalyst to reach the conclusion that I've already found it. It's not something that can be achieved externally; it always resides within us. We need only learn how to tap into it.

This is what I'm thinking as I complete the climb and take in the view of the temple before me. I carefully place the note into a small window on a building designed for prayer candles and memorials. It is an apt location for my father to discover my message. Gazing out at the breathtaking panorama of the monastery before me, I feel a deep sense of fulfillment—a fitting culmination of my father's request, yet a journey I vow to continue. It's a lifelong commitment, the grandest of promises to honour the memory of a loving parent.

My time in Bhutan gifts me with lasting insights into finding peace in my life. I learn to appreciate the beauty of simplicity and the significance of walking the

[opposite] Home in rural Punakha region
[page 64] Hidden temple in mountainside on Thimphu outskirts

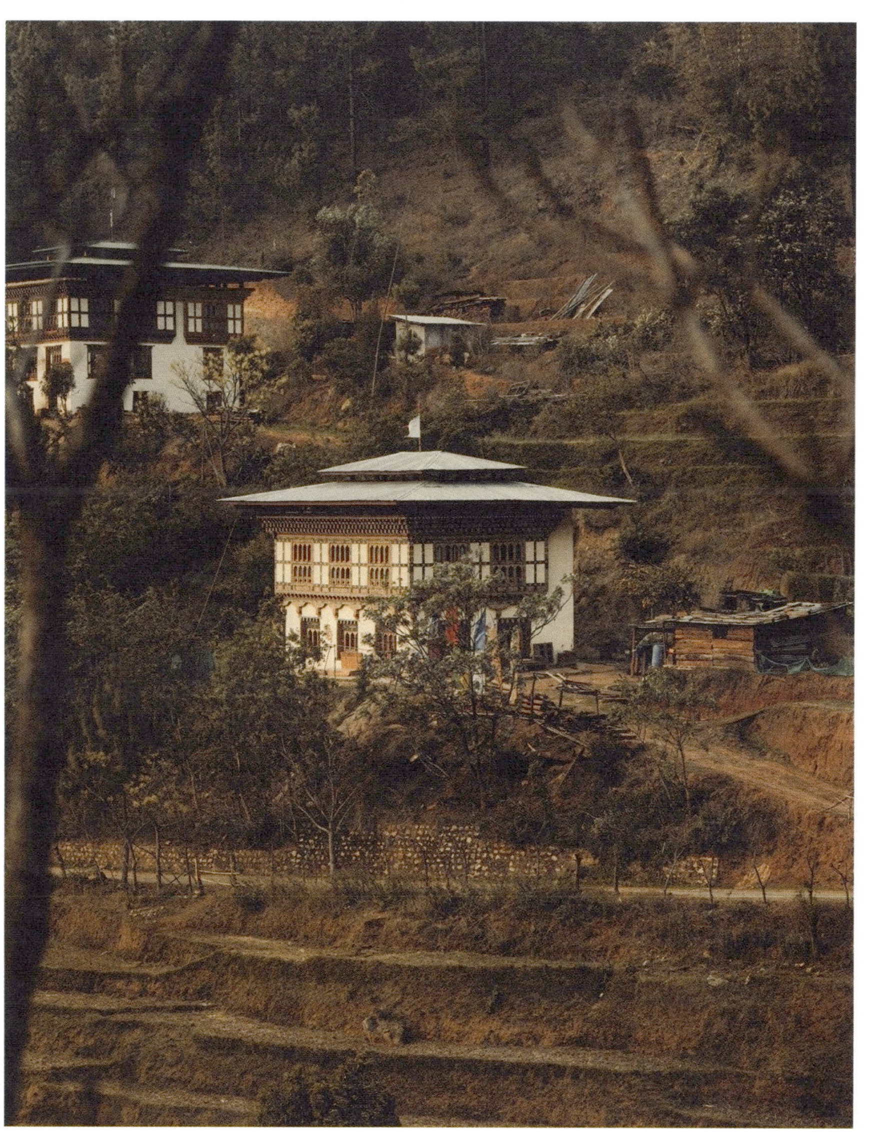

middle path in search of happiness. Moreover, I realize the power of shared values within a community. Just as Canadians are known for their kindness and friendliness, nurtured by the belief and emphasis placed upon those virtues, the Bhutanese prioritize happiness and wholeheartedly embrace it. Perhaps if we could collectively foster a shared vision of health, placing it at the forefront of our consciousness, it too could become a cherished value within our culture.

I came to Bhutan to witness firsthand the prioritization of happiness, and what I have discovered is that the choice to value it lies within each of us. However, there is undeniable strength and joy in being surrounded by others who share that same perspective—a community united in their pursuit of a common goal.

As I bid farewell to Bhutan, I carry with me a renewed sense of purpose, guided by the teachings of this hidden kingdom, and the enduring spirit of the Bhutanese people. The lessons learned among the majestic landscapes and warm-hearted souls have become a part of my very being, forever shaping my perspective. Finding happiness has been an exploration of myself, an introspection into what really matters, and a decluttering of what does not align. Happiness is not something you can find; it's the appreciation of what we already have.

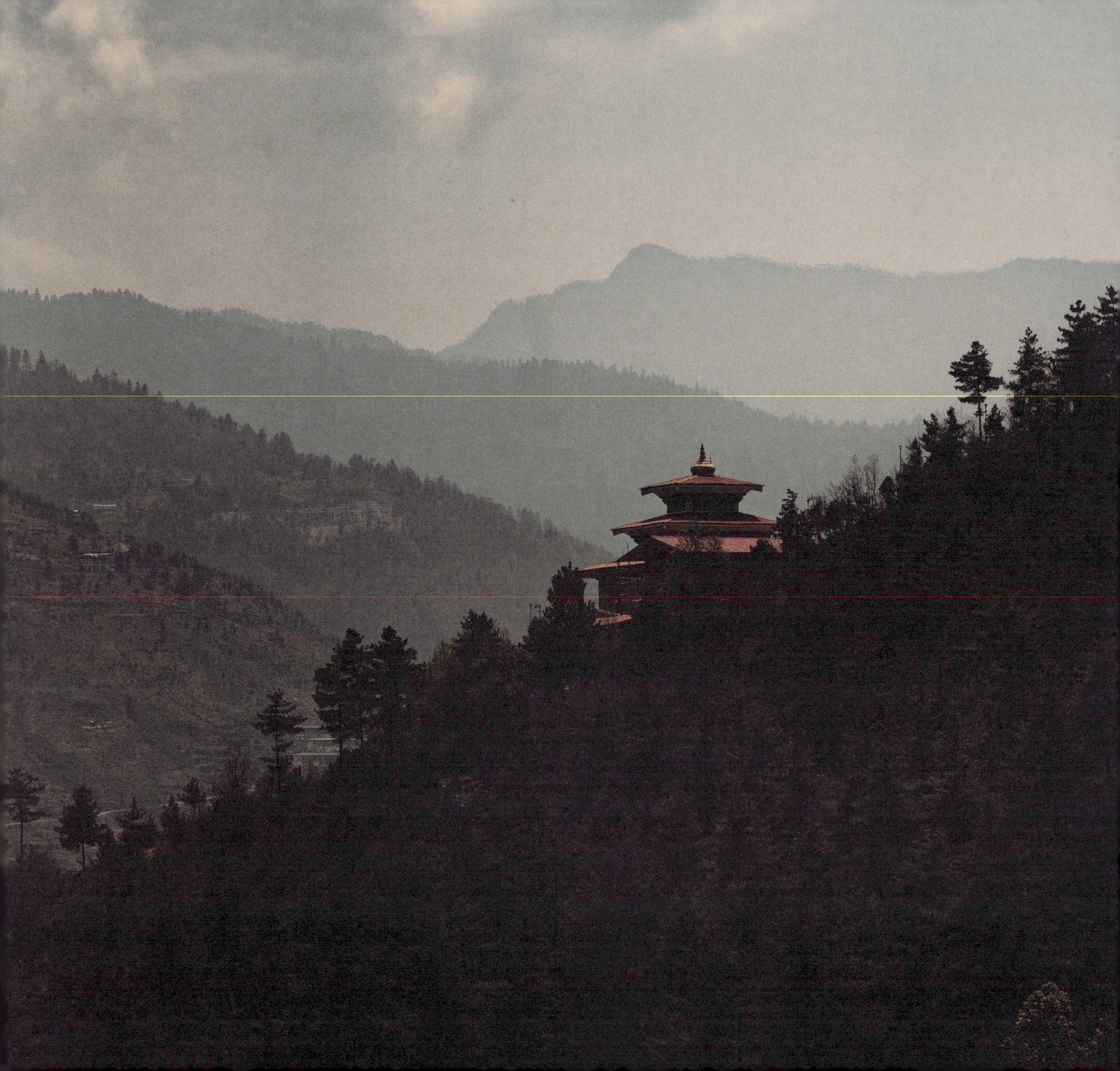

HEALING HAPPINESS: NURTURING WELL-BEING THROUGH BHUTAN'S GNH

These insights highlight how Bhutan's unique approach to Gross National Happiness (GNH) fosters well-being and happiness at the individual and societal levels.

HOLISTIC WELL-BEING: Bhutan's GNH framework emphasizes a comprehensive sense of well-being that goes beyond material wealth. It considers aspects such as mental health, cultural preservation, environmental sustainability, and community cohesion, creating a more balanced and fulfilling life experience for its citizens.

CULTURAL CONNECTION: GNH acknowledges the importance of cultural heritage and traditions in promoting happiness. Bhutan's emphasis on preserving its unique cultural identity enhances a sense of belonging and pride among its citizens, contributing to their overall happiness.

SHARED VALUES: The focus on common values like compassion, kindness, and spiritual growth in GNH encourages a sense of unity and shared purpose among Bhutanese citizens. This collective emphasis on positive values promotes social harmony and a strong sense of community, fostering happiness in daily life.

NATURAL HARMONY: Bhutan's respect for nature and the environment aligns with the philosophy of the GNH. The country's commitment to maintaining a carbon-neutral status and promoting sustainable practices allows its citizens to live in harmony with the natural world, contributing to a sense of well-being and interconnectedness.

MINDFUL PROGRESS: Instead of solely pursuing economic growth, GNH encourages a balanced approach to development. Bhutan's mindful progress considers the impact of development on well-being, ensuring that advancements benefit all aspects of life and don't compromise the happiness of its people.

FIND HAPPINESS WITHIN

By integrating these practices into your daily life, you can foster a positive and fulfilling experience that contributes to your overall happiness and well-being.

CULTIVATE GRATITUDE AND REFLECTION: Dedicate a few minutes each day to reflect on things you're grateful for. Write them down or simply think about them. This practice can shift your focus toward the positive aspects of your life and enhance your overall sense of happiness.

EMBRACE CONNECTION: Prioritize spending quality time with friends, family, and loved ones. Engage in meaningful conversations, listen attentively, and share your thoughts and feelings. Meaningful connections can bring joy and a sense of belonging.

DON'T SWEAT THE SMALL STUFF: While challenges are bound to exist, fixating on them can magnify their impact. Instead, adopt a solution-oriented mindset and resist the urge to excessively ruminate on difficulties. And don't take it personally when things go wrong. If you consistently apply this approach, it will foster resilience and well-being.

ENGAGE IN ACTS OF KINDNESS: Incorporate acts of kindness into your routine. This could be as simple as holding the door for someone, complimenting a colleague, or volunteering for a local charity. Acts of kindness not only benefit others but also contribute to your own sense of well-being.

PURSUE PERSONAL PASSIONS: Dedicate time to engage in activities that bring you genuine joy and satisfaction. Whether it's a creative hobby, playing a musical instrument, reading, or any other activity that resonates with you, pursuing your passions can provide a sense of accomplishment and happiness.

OUR HAPPINESS GUIDES

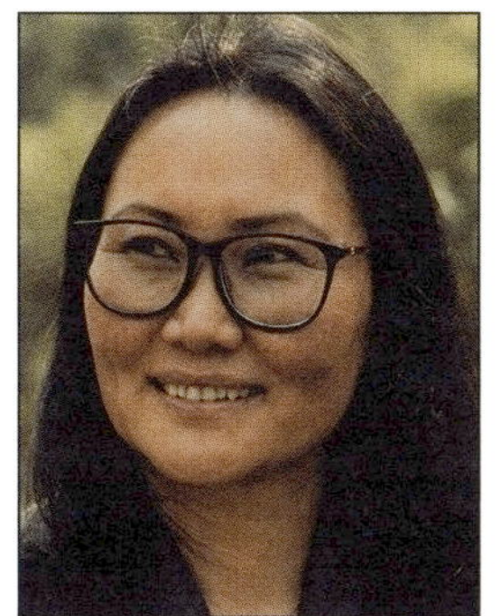

DR. CHENCHO LHAMU: A prominent figure in Bhutan's Department of Media and Democracy, Dr. Lhamu articulated the essence of Gross National Happiness (GNH), Bhutan's distinctive measure of progress. The multifaceted pillars and principles of GNH emphasize a holistic approach encompassing spiritual, social, cultural, and environmental dimensions. This comprehensive perspective, which Dr. Lhamu has been a major force behind, mirrors Bhutan's commitment to harmonizing progress with cultural heritage and sustainable resource management, demonstrating a nuanced understanding of societal advancement.

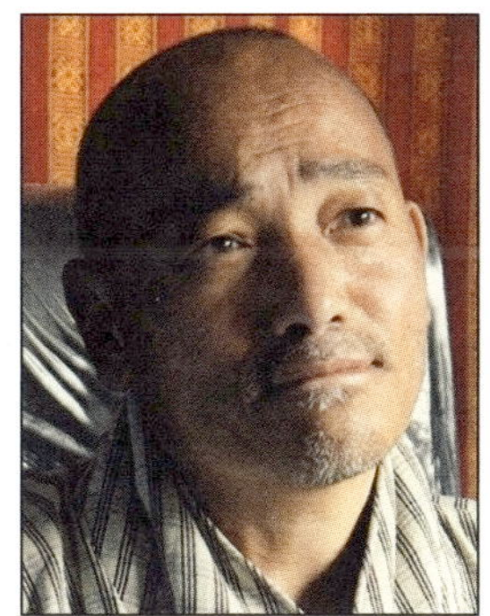

PRINCIPAL YOUNTEN JAMTSHO: Principal Jamtsho stands as a dedicated educator with a compelling vision. He places great emphasis on instilling the understanding of happiness' intrinsic value in the minds of young learners. He firmly believes that cultivating happiness early on is pivotal for their growth. He envisions an environment where learning, growth, and shared experiences intertwine to create lasting memories, fostering a foundation of happiness. With a commitment to nurturing their well-being, he actively engages students through sports, accomplishments, and a sense of belonging. As the head of Tashidingkha Central School in Punakha, Bhutan, Principal Jamtsho's influence goes beyond education—it extends into the realm of character building and the pursuit of lifelong happiness.

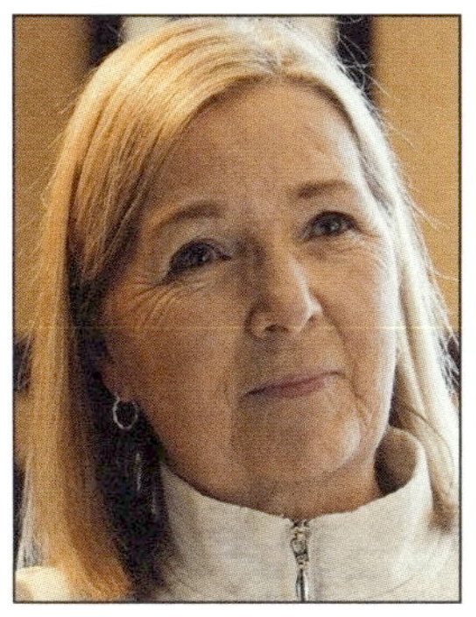

SHARON WAHL AND DR. JOHN WAHL: My parents' philosophy of "mining diamonds" offers invaluable insights into the nature of happiness. They taught me that life's true riches are found in the small, precious moments that often go unnoticed. Even in the face of my father's battle with cancer, they both emphasized the importance of cherishing every moment. My father's resilience in his cancer fight and my mother's battle with grief both serve as powerful reminders that the time we have is a gift to be embraced and celebrated. Their advice to not sweat the small stuff, and it's all small stuff, is valuable when facing the inevitable challenges in life.

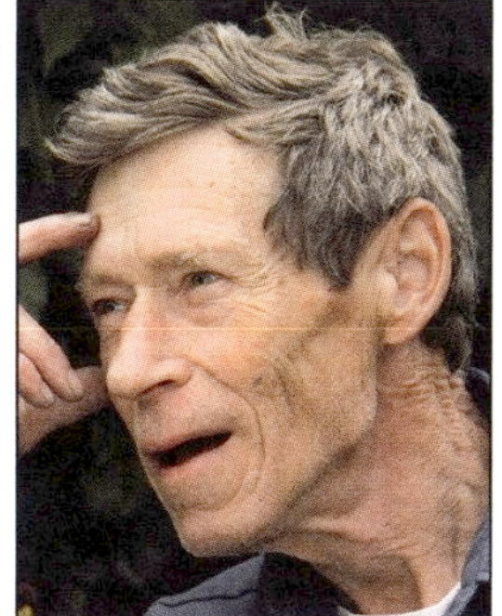

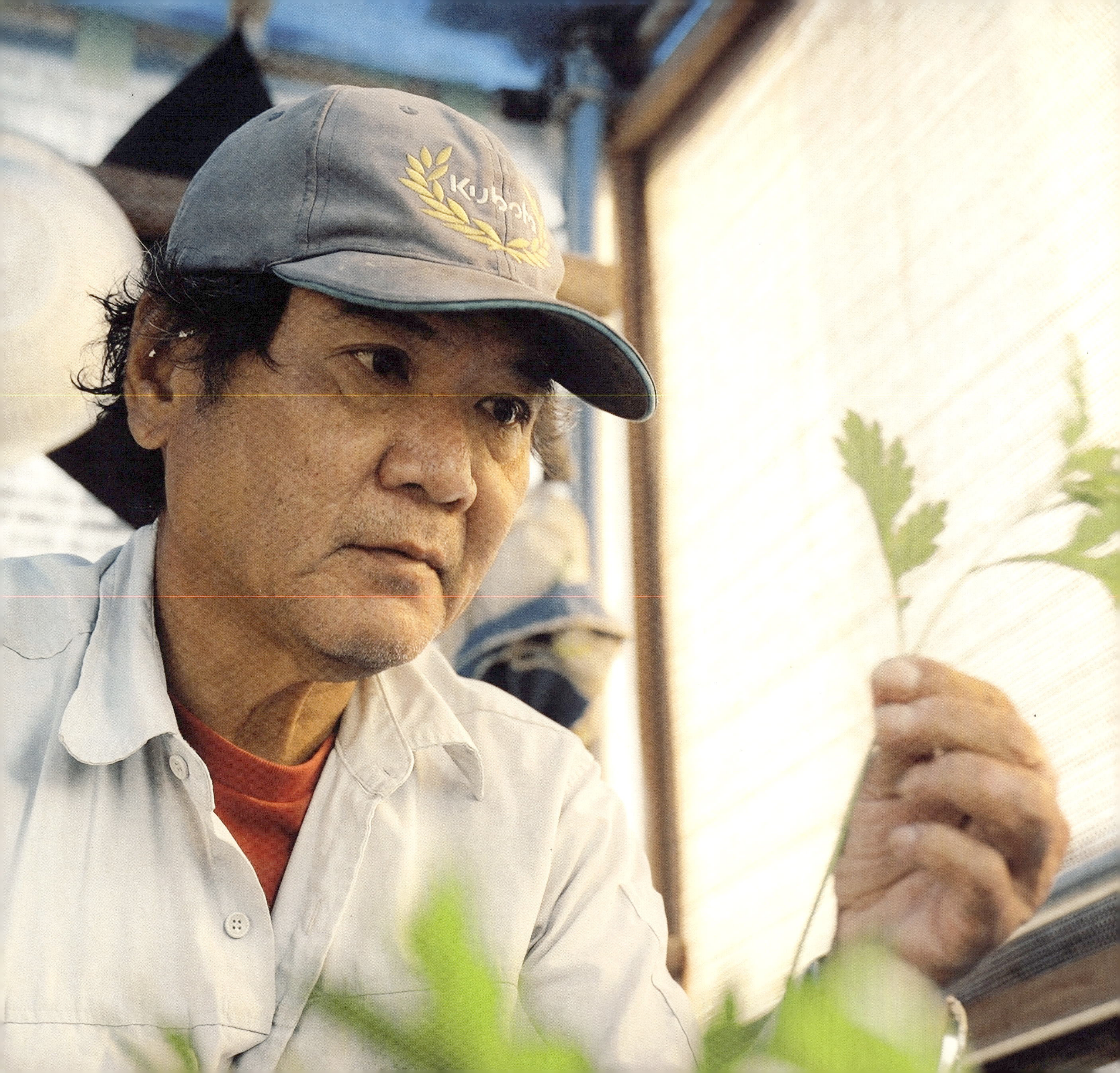

5

THE PURPOSE OF LIFE

On the remote island of Okinawa, stories of inspired spirits and enduring vitality come alive, unveiling the timeless essence of ikigai. Down winding roads, into bustling dojos, flourishing gardens, and quaint towns, I discover stories crafted with intention and infused with purpose

ISLAND OF THE IMMORTALS

I feel the gentle touch of the tropical sea breeze as I sit in my cozy rattan chair on the patio of the restaurant. Small flowers garnish the plate of rice and vegetables with specks of purple and yellow. The colourful cocktails, with pineapple and cherries sprouting from the glass, take me back to those vintage Elvis Presley movies set in the South Pacific. But instead of the familiar "Aloha," we are greeted with a cheerful "Konichiwa."

The pristine white sands and vibrant turquoise waters of Okinawa, Japan, paints a breathtaking picture in front of me, but it isn't just idyllic beaches that drew me here.

The allure of the Far East has always captivated me—its rich culture, ancient philosophies, and, more recently, the intriguing concept of ikigai. This has brought me to Okinawa, an island renowned for its long-living inhabitants. Here in this distant Blue Zone, I aim to unravel how passion, mission, vocation, and profession can intertwine to create a pattern of life filled with purpose and joy. It's about more than just living long—it's about how these lives are enriched by a fusion of purpose in life, the support of a close-knit community of lifelong friends called moai, and a special diet that emphasizes longevity foods.

Like all things, experiencing this lifestyle firsthand is entirely different from just reading about it. As I glance over my itinerary, I think about the meticulous months of planning that went into this trip. We faced language barriers, the unpredictable nature of interviewing the elderly, the strictest COVID-19 entry requirements in the world, and countless other challenges. I found my guide for the trip, Kumiko, through a media-specialized platform, and I was excited to meet her the next day. She'd packed my schedule with a lineup of interviews. She is simultaneously tense and excited, but I could tell she would be pressing to keep me on a tight schedule but also ensure that I enjoyed myself.

So, I set my phone down, sip my cocktail through its bamboo straw, and let myself get lost in the rhythm of the waves. Tomorrow, the real work begins.

[previous page] A belief in always growing
[opposite] Okinawa village from above

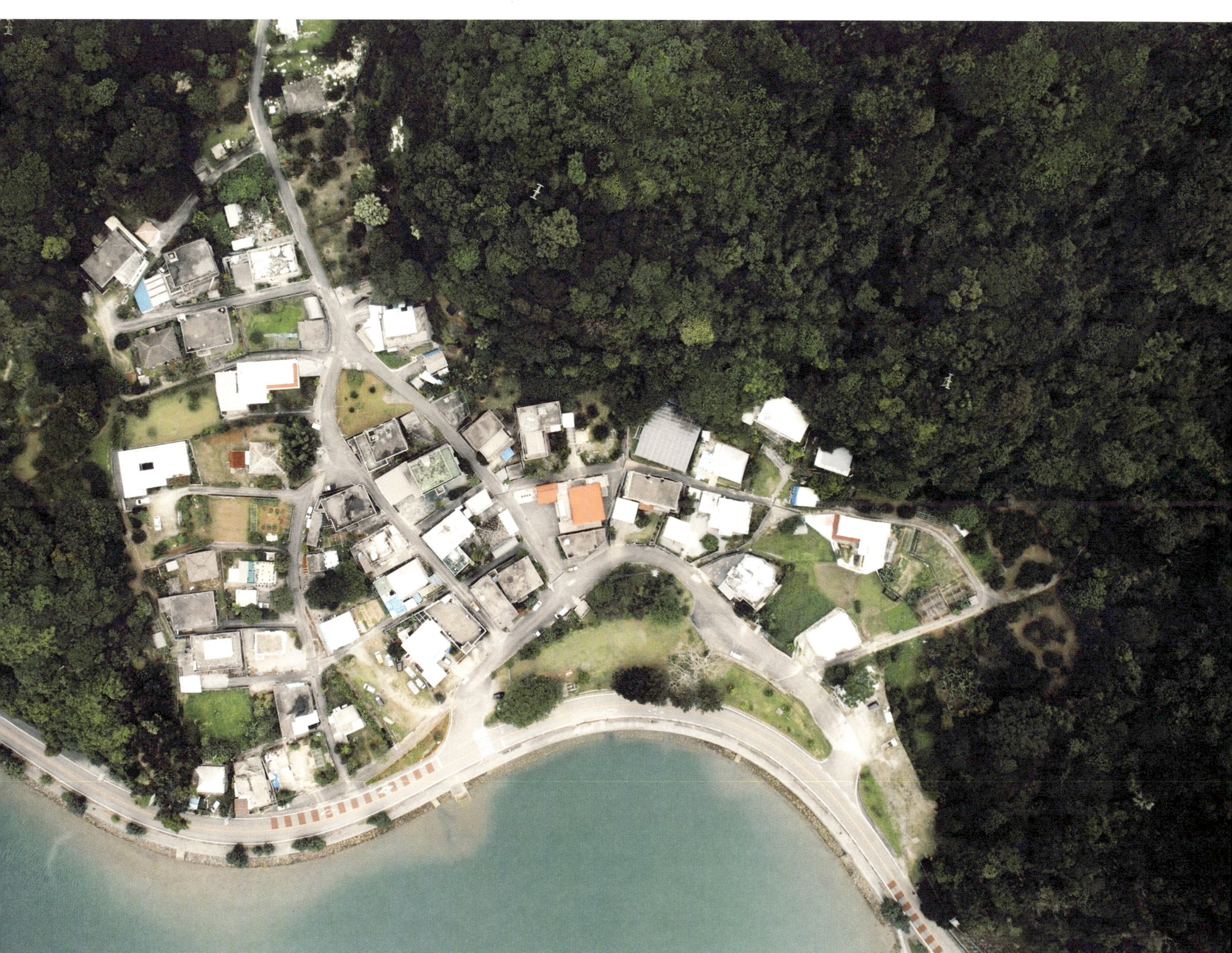

A NEW DAY

I'm up before dawn milling about in the dimly lit cabin I've rented as I collect my supplies for the day and daydream about coffee from the 7-Eleven down the road.

This is Day 26 of travel and my seventh country in a month. My spirits are high, but my energy is low until I remind myself where I am . . . paradise. The accommodation is a charming little wood cabin in the coastal farming village of Nanjo on the southwest coast of Okinawa. It masterfully blends the traditional with the contemporary. Sliding doors reveal straw rugs with plush mattresses, reminiscent of old-world Japan, and a rock-climbing wall hovers above a bed. The sunken kitchen, with counters flush with the main floor, allows for traditional seated dining.

Coffee in hand, I drive about fifteen minutes down the road to the rendezvous point identified by Kumiko. As soon as I park, an animated figure appears. Sporting a Strawberry Shortcake–like bonnet and a shoulder duffle, Kumiko eagerly waves some papers as she briskly approaches. Not willing to waste a moment, she begins speaking the instant I'm within earshot. Her warmth, energy, and infectious enthusiasm are just the boost I need after nearly a month on the road.

Often referred to as the "reason for being" or the essence that makes life truly worthwhile, the term ikigai melds *iki* (which means "to live") with *gai* (signifying "value" or "worth"). Originating in Japan, the concept of ikigai encapsulates the convergence of four primary elements:

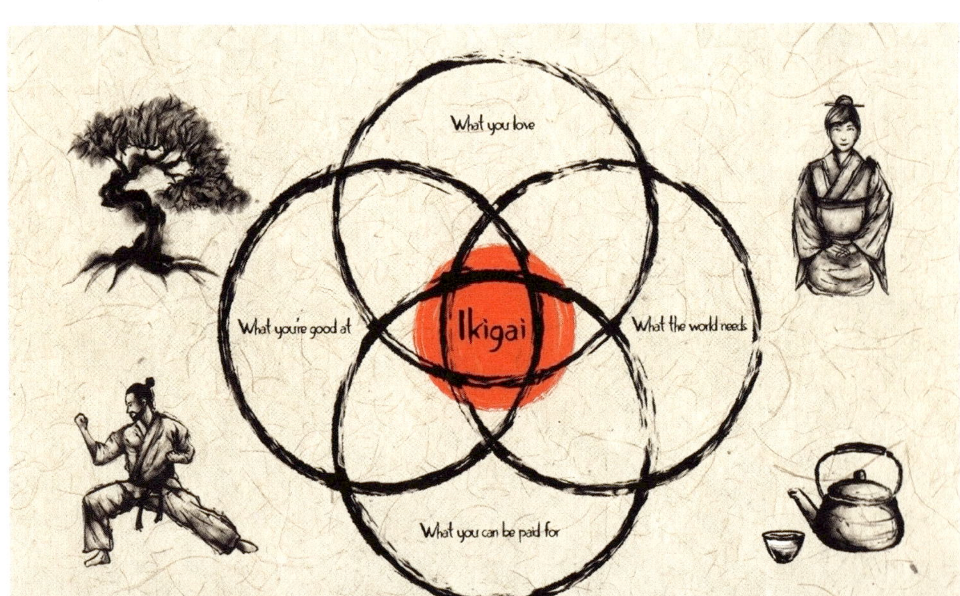

- **VOCATION:** The sphere where you apply your unique talents and abilities.
- **PROFESSION:** How you financially sustain yourself—essentially, your means of livelihood.
- **PASSION:** The things you're passionate about, those that energize you and bring joy.
- **MISSION:** Your larger purpose—what you believe adds value to the world or aids others.

The core belief behind ikigai is that when these four domains intersect, one achieves a profound sense of life satisfaction and joy. This alignment is thought to

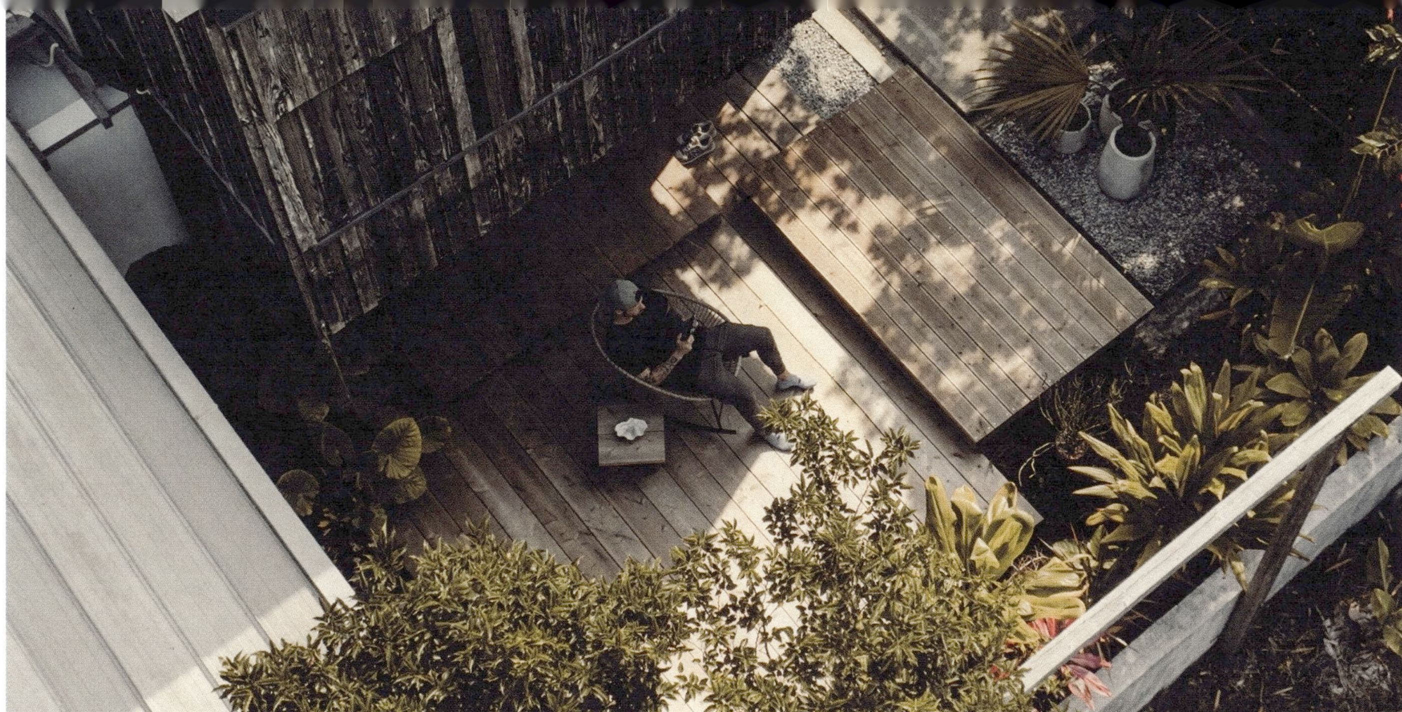

be a catalyst for a life that's not just longer but richer, healthier, and driven by purpose.

However, if even one of these elements is absent, there's a sense of imbalance. For instance, while passion invigorates us, it alone might not sustain us financially or necessarily benefit the greater good. A profession, though it provides financial stability, may require passion or the feeling that you're creating a benefit to the world. Vocation can be fulfilling and necessary, but it feels incomplete if it's devoid of joy or doesn't align with our innate strengths. And while a mission is undeniably essential, tackling it without the right tools or financial support can be demotivating—or even downright impossible.

Discovering one's ikigai involves introspection, self-awareness, and exploring the things that bring one joy and fulfillment. It is a process of finding balance and harmony between your inner desires and external contributions to society. People may find their ikigai through hobbies, work, relationships, or other meaningful activities that align with their passions, values, and talents.

I embarked on this journey to delve deeper into the concept of ikigai both for personal understanding and professional insight. I find the idea fascinating coming from a culture where the litany of life requirements, including get a good job, have a family, buy a house, and work for retirement drives adult decisions for many, regardless of whether it is indeed what they want.

Recently, I have been striving for things that resonate within me and shrinking from doing what does not fuel my passion. I wonder, have I been unintentionally seeking to align these four pivotal elements?

Hailing from a long line of geologists on my father's side, I imposed on my young self an expectation that I might tread that path. However, my parents always encouraged my passions. Consequently, I leaned into my mother's profession as a physical education teacher. The emerging field of kinesiology caught my attention, melding my interests in coaching, exercise, and science. While my father and grandfather held PhDs in geology, I carved out a different trajectory, one that felt tailor-made for me. It was as if I was cruising on my personal Autobahn, a clear path without bounds.

I've always considered myself fortunate to have found such fulfilling work, a sentiment both my parents echoed in their careers. Over the years, I've come to appreciate that their guidance was far more intentional than I ever realized. This retrospective insight underscores the wisdom that older generations offer, and it was this very concept that drew me to Okinawa.

Perhaps I was looking for justification for my unconventional life or a citation I could reference if confronted by traditionalists. I was curious about how a culture could plant the concept of meaningful purpose into its core and watch it grow to create a rich, long life for its citizens.

[opposite] Ikigai—the philosophy of finding purpose
[above] Cabin on the coast

VOCATION: SAVOURING LIFE

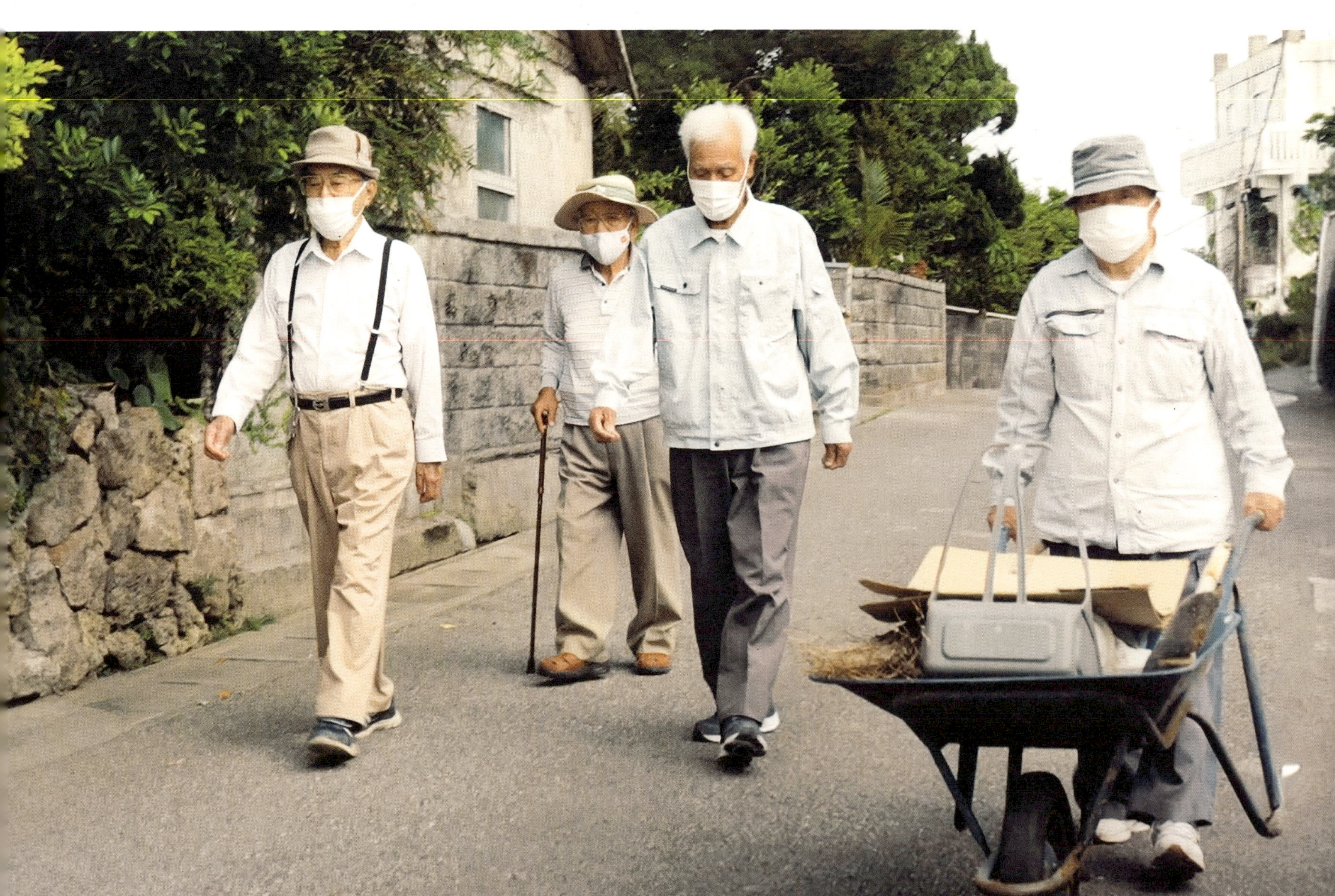

My first stops are designed to help me understand the nature of longevity foods on this tiny island. Foods like sweet potatoes, fresh vegetables, rice, small amounts of meats and fish, and other unfamiliar ingredients are staples in the Okinawan diet. These foods have been credited in cookbooks dedicated to health, in documentaries, and in popular media as a secret to living a longer, healthy life. Okinawa's traditional diet isn't a vegetarian diet; there are small amounts of pork and fish woven in, but it emphasizes moderation and foods high in fibre and carbohydrates. Our teacher for the day will be the chef at a well-known longevity food café. She prepares foods that are being lost in time for her community. In doing so, she satisfies both the goal of doing something the world needs as well as doing something that can sustain her financially.

This is the essence of vocation, and I'm eager to taste these magical foods I've read so much about.

But first, I want to see where much of the local produce comes from, so Kumiko takes me on a stroll through a slice of Okinawa's farm-to-table tradition.

When we exit our vehicle at a local farm, we're greeted by a farmer standing in a small plot surrounded by a patchwork of fields. His pristine white minitruck is parked on a slope adjacent to his cultivated land. With a gesture, he beckons us to join him as he picks vegetables destined for the market: a medley of sweet potatoes, carrots, radishes, and okra, all neatly resting in his modest wheelbarrow. Together with his colleague, he expertly cleans and packages the harvest into small containers, which we assist in loading onto the truck. The operation, though seemingly simple, is rich in yield, and the farmer's pride is evident in his beaming smile as he passionately shares details about each vegetable.

Even when Kumiko, my translator, steps away to take a call, the farmer continues his enthusiastic narration in Japanese. While I can't comprehend the words, I reciprocate his enthusiasm with nods and smiles, wanting to convey my admiration for his work and skill in farming.

When Kumiko returns, she informs me that my next destination is an hour's drive away, and my upcoming host is eagerly anticipating our arrival. With bows and handshakes, I express my gratitude to our hospitable farmer. Then, we hop into our SUV to journey to the other side of the island.

The journey to the village of Ogimi is one of gradual transformation. The urban cacophony of the capital of Naha gives way to a serene pastoral landscape, and the tempo of life visibly slows. We drive along beautiful coastlines where surfers dot the reef in an uncrowded peace. The road winds around small bays with golden beaches framing giant limestone monoliths, each with its own jungle on top. The area is noticeably pristine, free from litter and without a speck of graffiti anywhere. As we enter the village, tiny traditional Japanese houses comprise the view, their wooden verandas, and stone roofs reminders of the village's history. In the distance, the shimmering waters of the ocean promise stories of their own and wrap the bay with golden sand.

Nestled amidst this backdrop is Emiko Kinjo's pride and joy, Emi no Mise. From a distance, the restaurant exudes a rustic charm: Its wooden facade, aged gracefully under the Okinawan sun, stands out against the emerald expanse of surrounding fields. Terracotta pots with blooming flowers line the entrance, and the soft chime of wind bells adds a melodic welcome.

Upon arriving, we're met by Emiko herself, her face crinkling into a warm smile that instantly feels familiar. Her hands, stained with the earth, hint at a morning spent in the garden. With a gesture of invitation, she leads us toward the field, her gait steady and sure.

The garden is a picture of vibrant hues: greens, purples, yellows, and reds. The sun casts a subtle glow, illuminating Emiko's simple dress and apron as she inspects her vegetable patch. Her fingers pass over each leaf, almost as if communicating with the plants. She hums a soft tune—a traditional Okinawan melody, perhaps—as she works, plucking vegetables with the precision of an artist selecting colours for a masterpiece.

And then she begins to chat, speaking of each vegetable's significance, flavour profile, and place in Okinawan cuisine. We trail behind, Kumiko interpreting as she goes, captivated by Emiko's knowledge and the palpable connection she shares with her land.

The journey from garden to kitchen is short but transformative. Emiko's workspace is a juxtaposition of traditional and modern. Pots and pans hang from wooden beams; stone mortars sit alongside sleek kitchen gadgets. But it's Emiko's dance between them that truly mesmerizes me. Her culinary ritual unfolds like a well-rehearsed ballet: She washes, chops, stirs, and tastes with a grace that makes it all seem effortless.

The aroma that fills the kitchen is intoxicating. Herbs and spices mingle with the fresh scent of harvested vegetables, creating an olfactory experience that promises a feast for the senses. As Emiko orchestrates this culinary performance, her dedication to her craft—her vocation—is evident. Every move and every gesture are imbued with purpose.

Sitting down to dine at Emi no Mise after witnessing the journey from garden to plate is a memorable experience. Each bite tells a story, not just of Okinawan tradition but of Emiko's unwavering commitment to her community and her vocation. The experience becomes a tale of nature, tradition, and the artistry of a woman dedicated to her craft.

As the last bites are savoured and the lingering flavours fade, Emiko settles beside me, a pot of traditional Okinawan tea in hand. The gentle steam rising from the cup is comforting as she begins to share her story.

"Emi no Mise is not just a café," she begins, her eyes reflecting the years of passion she has poured into it. "It's a beacon, a testament to the traditions of Ogimi. It's my life's work." She explains that many years ago, she noticed a gradual shift away from the dietary staples that had sustained the village for generations. Younger generations were leaning toward modern diets, and with that shift, age-old recipes and culinary wisdom were slowly fading.

It isn't just about food for Emiko. It's about identity, heritage, and health. Ogimi, known for its high concentration of centenarians, holds secrets in its traditional diet—a balance of nutrients, flavours, and nature's goodness. Emiko's endeavour with Emi no Mise is to bridge the gap between generations, to ensure that the wisdom of the elderly isn't lost but passed down, preserved, and celebrated.

Her commitment goes beyond the confines of her café. Emiko initiated programs where the elderly could share their knowledge with the youth, facilitating sessions on farming techniques, vegetable cultivation, and traditional cooking methods. This has not only fostered community bonding but ensured that the old traditions of Ogimi have a future.

For Emiko, this isn't just how she makes a living—it is her ikigai, her reason for being. By revitalizing and championing the traditional diet, she provides the community with more than just sustenance; she gifts them longevity and a sense of belonging. Watching young and old sit side by side, laughing, learning, and dining together, is the reward that adds meaning to her life.

Emiko's gaze drifts toward the window, capturing the bright sun that bathes her garden in a golden hue. "When I plant a seed," she shares, "I'm not just growing food. I'm nurturing hope. Hope for a future where our traditions thrive, where every meal tells a story, and where every story brings us closer as a community."

The afternoon winds down, but the resonance of Emiko's words remain engrained to this day. How lucky is it to feel inspired, to preserve a tradition and to speak about it with such conviction. Her life's work is a testament to the power of purpose. In the union of food, tradition, and community, she has found her true calling, illuminating the lives of those around her, one meal, one story at a time.

PROFESSION: MASTERING PURPOSE

Upon arriving at the dojo—a meeting hall, typically where martial arts are practised—I can sense the ancient history embedded within its walls. My guide through this portion of the journey of discovery is none other than Masahiro Nakamoto, an esteemed 10th dan black belt master, still strong and agile at the age of eighty-eight. His presence is magnetic, commanding respect without saying a word. Although short in stature, standing just above five feet tall, he radiates the presence of a giant. His build is sturdy and strong, his snow-white beard perfectly trimmed. His eyes are wise and calm yet astute and interrogating, and he exudes an aura wrapped in warmth and respect. Coming into that commanding presence, I immediately sense that he will be one of the most interesting individuals I have ever met.

The dojo's atmosphere is serene and filled with respect and discipline. At the entrance stands a museum that details the rich history of Kobudo, a martial art that uniquely incorporates weapons into its techniques. The relics and artifacts tell tales of warriors, battles, and the intricacies of the craft. He shows me canes with hidden blades, umbrellas that are swords, and jewellery with poison spikes, one after another. Almost embarrassingly, I catch my Western mind remembering that Kobudo was the martial art of choice in my favourite childhood show, *Teenage Mutant Ninja Turtles*.

As we tour the museum, Nakamoto sensei elaborates on the various weapons used in Kobudo, emphasizing the bō, sai, eku, tonfa, suruchin, tekko, and kama. Each weapon, he explains, is an extension of one's body and soul. He tells me that in different periods of Okinawa's history, especially during the rule of mainland Japan, there were bans on carrying or using weapons. These bans led the Okinawans to adapt everyday farming tools as improvised weapons for self-defence. For instance, the kama (a sickle) and the nunchaku (rice flail) are both agricultural tools that were repurposed for martial arts use.

Having soaked in the history, we move to the heart of the dojo, where Nakamoto sensei has a unique demonstration planned for me. With a ten-kilogram sledgehammer in hand, he lifts his gi to reveal a hardened shin. Then he motions to quiet the room to ensure total silence and, picking up the heavy mallet, strikes his shin with force. The sound echoes throughout the dojo, yet he stands unphased. He then places the sledgehammer on the ground and, with a swift kick to the side of the handle, sends it bouncing back up so he can effortlessly catch it.

I can't help but smile. This is the first time I have ever met a true master.

After the bone-crunching demonstration, it's time for the nunchaku lesson. The master, in his wisdom, has me don a traditional gi, allowing me to at least feel like I'm an actual participant. His teaching style is a testament to his character: patience incarnate, unwavering dedication, and an innate ability to inspire.

The intricacies of the nunchaku become immediately apparent as we dive into our lesson. My initial attempts are clumsy, and the sensei has to demonstrate the moves multiple times, breaking down each motion to ensure I grasp the concept. His son, also a world champion, is the one on whom I practise my takedowns. Despite his status as a master, he approaches the exercise with lightheartedness, allowing me to execute slow takedowns on him, always

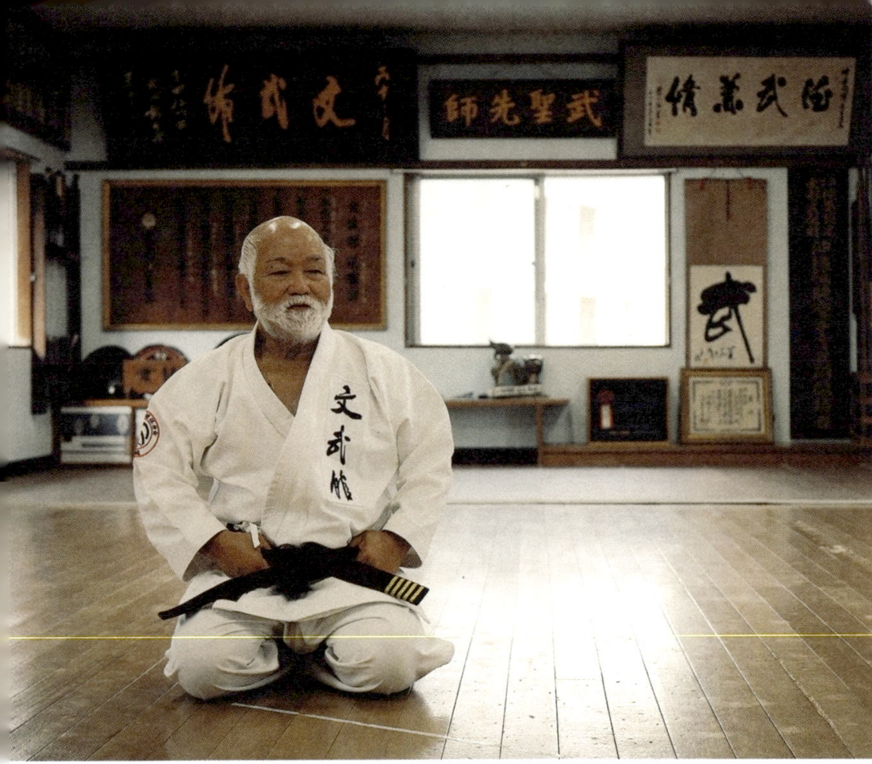

with a supportive smile. Through this practice, I realize just how intricate and complicated Kobudo is: It's a dance of the mind and body, demanding years, if not a lifetime, to truly master.

By the session's end, I have managed to muster a handful of quick moves, winning some memorable nods of approval from the sensei. We then try to string these together into patterns. These sequences are fundamental in grading and standardizing skills in Kobudo. As I move in "tandem" with some of the world's best, I feel an over-whelming sense of gratitude. To learn, even if just the basics, side by side with such masters is an honour I'll cherish forever.

When I take a break, Nakamoto sensei shares some of his wisdom with me.

"Kobudo," he begins, "is not just about wielding weapons. It's about treasuring traditional techniques, protecting our lives, and building good relationships with people. This discipline has added meaning and purpose to my life, offering both physical and mental health benefits." His words emphasize how Kobudo is not only a martial art but a way of life, a path to holistic well-being. He likens practising Kobudo to eating rice—a daily habit one must not miss lest they lose themselves.

The conversation then veers toward his years of teaching. Over six decades, he has taught thousands, directly or indirectly, through his branch dojos across the globe. Yet, despite his global acclaim, his humility is striking. To him, every student is a unique individual deserving of dedicated guidance.

As the day comes to an end, the sensei leads me to a small section of his home. It is an art gallery hidden under the dojo. His paintings adorn the walls and are magnificent. He has a beautiful portrait of his late wife, whom he very clearly adored, and ink paintings of bullfighters, samurai, and dramatic nature scenes. It appears his mastery extends to the arts as a gentler side is revealed in this sanctuary. He sits and wets a quill in ink, opening a copy of his book, *The Martial Arts and Art*, a testament to his dual mastery of both Kobudo and traditional sumi-e ink painting. He places a stone on the corner of the book to leave it open as the ink dries and motions for me to move toward the table where a large scroll lies wrapped with a silk ribbon.

"For you," he says and bows.

Astonished, I ask if I can open it, and he nods in approval. I pull the delicate ribbon and lift the scroll, carefully letting the banner roll open. Kumiko moves close as the Japanese writing on the scroll is revealed. "It is Bushido," she exclaims, "the way of the warrior." It is a symbol of the life lessons imparted within this dojo.

Accepting this scroll, I am overwhelmed by an incredible sense of honour. This is not merely a gift; Kumiko explains that it's a sacred passage of wisdom, a mark of respect signifying that the sensei sees me worthy to bear this deep philosophical inheritance. The scroll symbolizes the virtues of Bushido: honour, discipline, loyalty, and the sensei's recognition of my potential to embody these principles in life.

Today, in the presence of Masahiro Nakamoto, I didn't just witness the essence of Kobudo. I was privy to a master's life journey, one that was deeply intertwined with passion, discipline, and a relentless pursuit of mastery. It is clear that his profession is not just a career choice; it's his ikigai, his reason for being.

[above] Sensie Nakamoto—The martial arts and art

PASSION: CULTIVATING MEANING

Nestled in the picturesque backdrop of Ogusuku, meticulously curated gardens bloom as silver-haired men in matching blue overalls mill about, forming an organized team of purpose.

The energy of this place is palpable. Octogenarians fervently nurture the community gardens, their passion evident in every petal and leaf. These men are artists, with nature as their canvas. In their hands, dull patches of roadside metamorphose into pleasing visions. The camaraderie they share, honed over years of togetherness, shines through their lighthearted banter and the tales they recount. It becomes clear to me: Gardening isn't just a hobby. It's their ikigai, a shared purpose that binds them to their community and each other. Now retired, many channel their love of the outdoors into this purpose. The creativity of a life unburdened by a career unfolds in the brilliance and thoughtfulness of their gardens, adding immeasurable value to their communities. Butterflies float by, beckoned by colourful flowers and gorgeous green walls of leaves. I can picture working-age adults driving by their gardens, inspired by what creativity, unencumbered by deadlines, can produce.

The gardeners graciously allow me to assist in their labour of love. Their pace is brisk, their movements well practised. As we transition from one garden to the next, they generously impart their wisdom, guiding me in planting and pruning. Passing a tree, a fragrant scent captures my attention, leading me to spot where orchids have been expertly grafted onto their branches and trunks. This masterful botany yields incredible flowers. So exquisite are these creations that I'm told they sell them for charity, gathering funds for their collective endeavours.

The town, acknowledging the gardeners' passion, backs them wholeheartedly.

After an hour of surprisingly fast-paced labour, we pause for a break. We settle under a blossoming tree's shade. Warm cups of tea and cool glasses of water circulate. Here, surrounded by their curated natural embrace, the gardeners share stories of their friendship. Ranging in age from their late sixties to well into their nineties, many have shared bonds for over half a century. Their stories craft a vivid portrayal of moai—the Okinawan notion of lifelong friends united for mutual support. Their connections through friendship and love for gardening have transformed the entire town into a picturesque and pleasing community. This extends beyond the roots of the plants and flowers; it's their bond, their shared memories, and their commitment to their neighbours that genuinely illustrate their moai.

These gardens thrive not just from soil and sun but from the mutual purpose and respect that those who tend them bear for each other, echoing the interconnectedness and harmony foundational to the Okinawan way of life. Their collective ikigai manifests in every garden they tend and offers a lesson for us all: Our most significant accomplishments come when we are freed from the confines of working for money to revel in pursuits infused with passion.

MISSION: INSPIRING HEALTH

Found woven into the historical and scenic beauty of Okinawa lies an enchanting facet of its culture: the celebration of life and graceful aging. In the town of Kitanakagusuku, this is honoured annually through a unique wellness pageant.

My journey brings me to this closely knit town of white buildings and winding roads, where I meet the reigning Miss Kitanakagusuku. At eighty-eight, Kikue Taira—or Ms. K, as everyone fondly calls her—is the epitome of grace, vitality, and tenacity. Sitting poised for our conversation, her impeccable posture and manicured appearance impress me immediately. In her, I see the very essence of ikigai, a living testament to why a healthy lifestyle is foundational for a fulfilling life.

She eagerly delves into her daily routines, highlighting her dedication to wellness. Every Tuesday, Ms. K finds herself dancing and exercising in a communal space, while monthly doctor visits ensure she remains in peak health. As she describes her daily walks to the sea, I nod in agreement with our shared health values.

To supplement her outdoor activities, Ms. K has designed stretches she practises on her bed, focusing on her lower back and legs. She proudly demonstrates her ability to touch beyond her toes, placing her palms flat on the ground. Her regular bicycle rides, sometimes spanning over eight kilometres to a shopping mall, not only maintain her physique but also lend her a youthful aura, which she wears like a badge of honour.

Her diet, primarily traditional Japanese cuisine, comprises a mix of vegetables with a touch of meat. This nutritional balance and her unwavering commitment to exercise might be her fountain of youth. And while she shields herself with sunblock, she's also mindful of the sun's gift of vitamin D, which is crucial for robust bones.

Reflecting on her participation in the pageant, she speaks of how the Atta Community Association nudged her to join. Initially hesitant, she yielded to the incessant praises and encouragement of friends who saw her true vitality.

As she recounts all this, I can't help but be in awe of this inspiring figure. Beyond her routines, her spirit is what captivates me the most. Her joys range from dancing to mingling with the community's youth, but what truly warms her heart is seeing her children prosper. The community's regard for Ms. K is palpable, and I'm struck by the contrast in our treatment of seniors back home. I'm reminded of the value and wisdom we often overlook and the societal conditioning that nudges our elderly toward a subdued existence. The realization dawns: We might have much to learn from the East in our reverence for the elderly. After all, ikigai doesn't have an expiry date.

As I leave Kitanakagusuku, Ms. K's narrative serves as a potent reminder: True beauty and wellness go beyond daily choices; they encompass finding joy, purpose, and community in our lives.

I head to the beach for a final stroll beside the waves, taking a page out of Ms. K's book. This voyage has been transformative, underscoring the importance of living in sync with nature, purpose, and community—the very heart of ikigai.

The Kobudo master, with his unwavering discipline, exemplified the power of continuous learning and adaptability. The communal gardeners, tending their plots with shared commitment, reflected the island's spirit of unity and collaboration. The insightful chef highlighted the importance of nurturing through

[opposite] The farms of Nanjo, Okinawa

sustenance, reminding us that food is more than just nutrition—it's a testament to tradition. And the reigning Miss Kitanakagusuku, with her vibrant energy, epitomized the essence of aging with grace and vitality.

Yet, beyond these individuals, it was the collective integrity of values in Okinawa that left an indelible mark. The society here didn't just respect their seniors, they revered them—viewing them not as fading stars but as guiding lights, their brilliance forged through years of experiences and wisdom.

Reflecting on my time here, I realize health isn't just about the steps we take or the food we eat. It's found in the moments of joy we embrace, the passions we chase, and the connections we forge. True health melds the physical, mental, spiritual, and communal.

As my plane takes off, leaving behind the beautiful anomaly that is Okinawa, a deep sense of gratitude wells within me: gratitude for the lessons learned, the stories shared, and the philosophy embraced. Okinawa was more than a destination; it was an invitation to find my ikigai, a lifelong discovery of purpose. In the journey of life, the quest remains singular—to find a reason for being and, in doing so, live a life truly worth living.

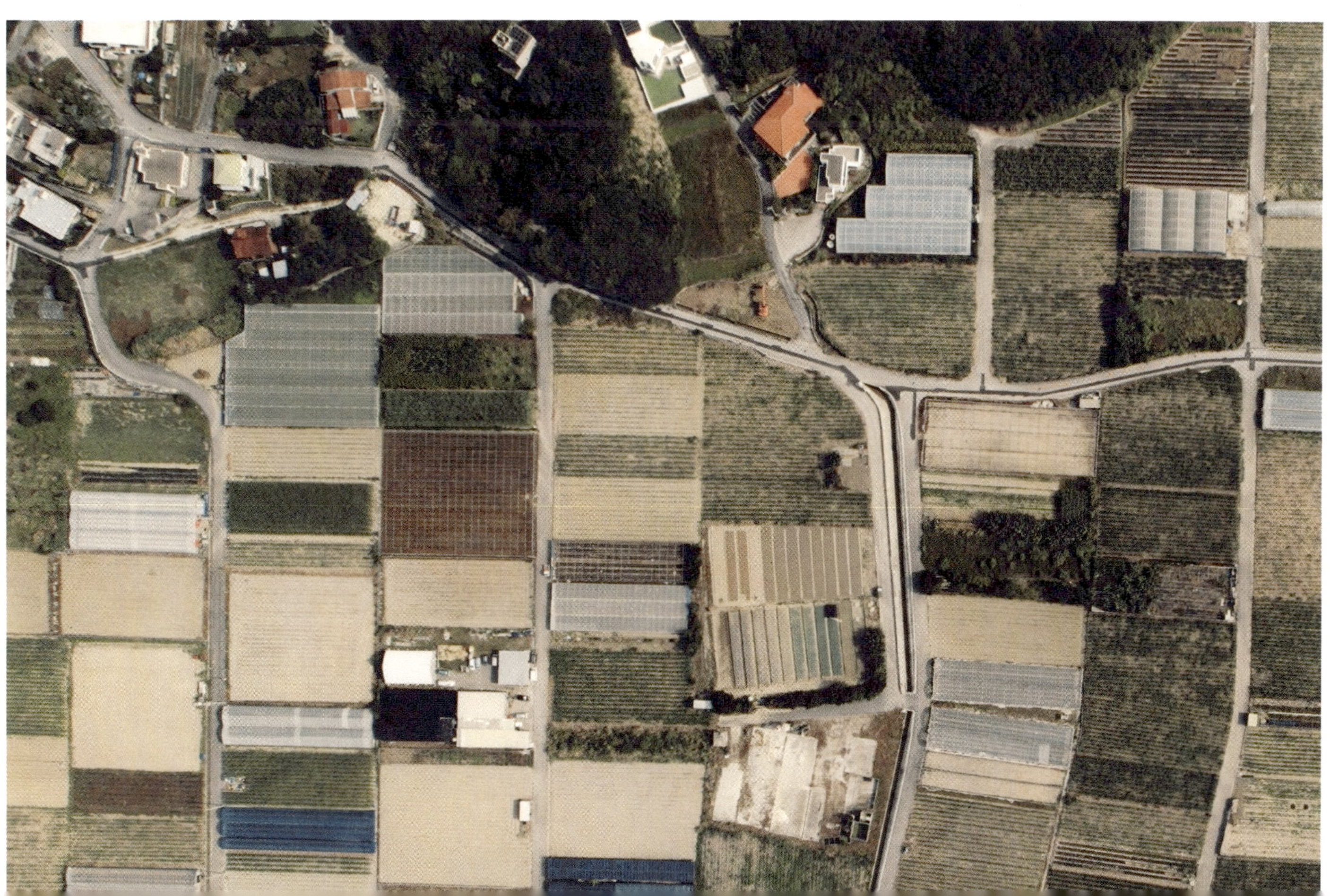

FIND IKIGAI AND LIVE A PURPOSEFUL LIFE

LEARN AND ADAPT CONTINUOUSLY: Seek knowledge and be open to change. This growth mindset can guide you closer to your purpose.

CULTIVATE COMMUNITY: Surround yourself with like-minded individuals who support and share your passions, fostering a sense of unity and collective purpose.

SERVE WITH LOVE: Identify how you can uplift others. True satisfaction often comes from serving others.

EMBRACE AGING: Live with passion regardless of age. Never let age deter you from pursuing what you love.

BUILD PILLARS OF HEALTH: Focus on mental, physical, and spiritual wellness. This balance is essential to living your best life.

REVERE EXPERIENCE AND WISDOM: Value the wisdom of seniors or those with more experience and how they can offer valuable insights into purpose and meaning.

REFLECT ON JOY AND PASSION: Consistently ponder what genuinely makes you happy, what activities make time fly, and where you find joy. These are often indicators of where your ikigai might lie.

THE ELDERS WHO TAUGHT US

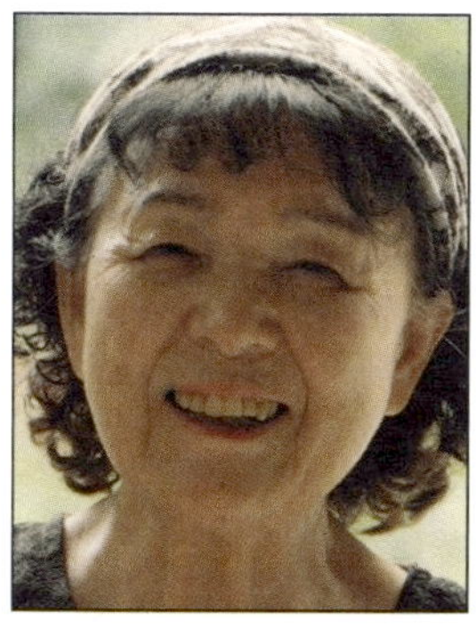

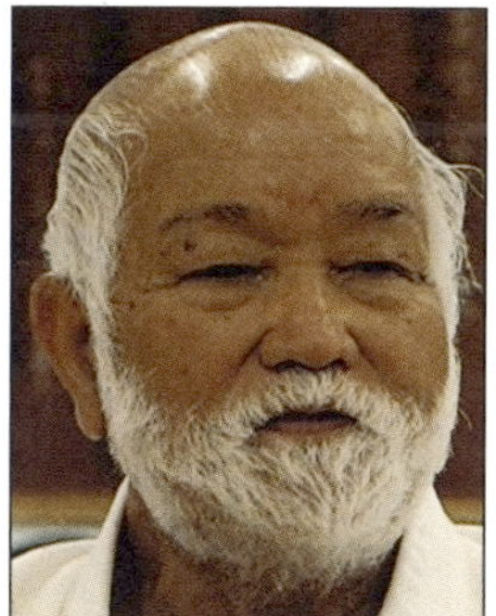

VOCATION—THE CHEF: The chef illustrates the depth of meaning in nourishing others. Through her culinary expertise, she reminds us that food is not just sustenance but an act of love and care. Her vocation transcends simply preparing meals; it's about connecting with and nurturing her community. She embodies the idea that true fulfill-ment in one's vocation comes from service and connection to others.

PROFESSION—THE KOBUDO MASTER: The Kobudo master exemplifies dedication and disci-pline in mastering his art. His unwavering commitment to the martial art craft teaches the importance of continuous learning and adapt-ability. He embodies the idea that expertise comes not just from skill but from a deep love for one's craft. Through his journey, we understand that one's profession can be a lifelong pursuit fuelled by passion and respect for a discipline.

PASSION—THE COMMUNAL GARDENERS: The communal gardeners of Okinawa empha-size the beauty of collective effort and mutual respect. Their shared gardens are not just about cultivation but about community, symbolizing the Okinawan ethos of unity and collaboration. Their passion shows that meaningful work arises from shared goals and commitments and that nurturing some-thing together can strengthen bonds and create lasting value.

MISSION—MISS KITANAKAGUSUKU: Miss Kitanakagusuku, with her radiant spirit, showcases that age is no barrier to living with zeal. Her daily routines, from exercising to dancing, highlight a life of purpose and joy. She underscores the significance of maintaining physical and mental wellness, irrespective of age. Through her, we learn that mission can be a constant companion, fuelling our days with energy and purpose.

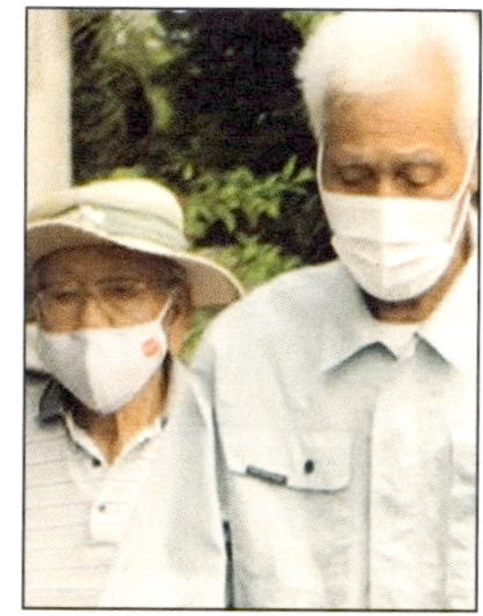

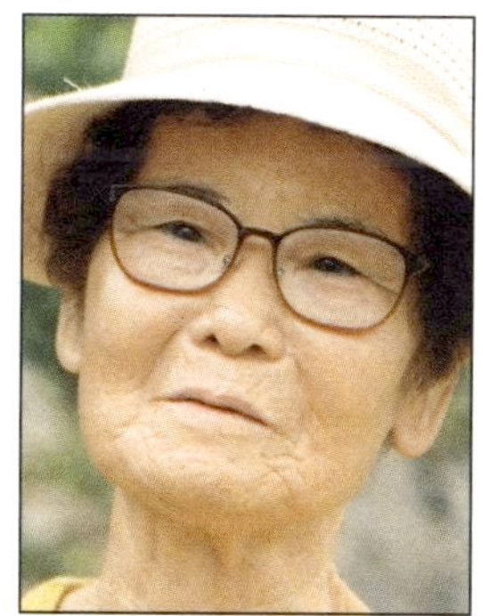

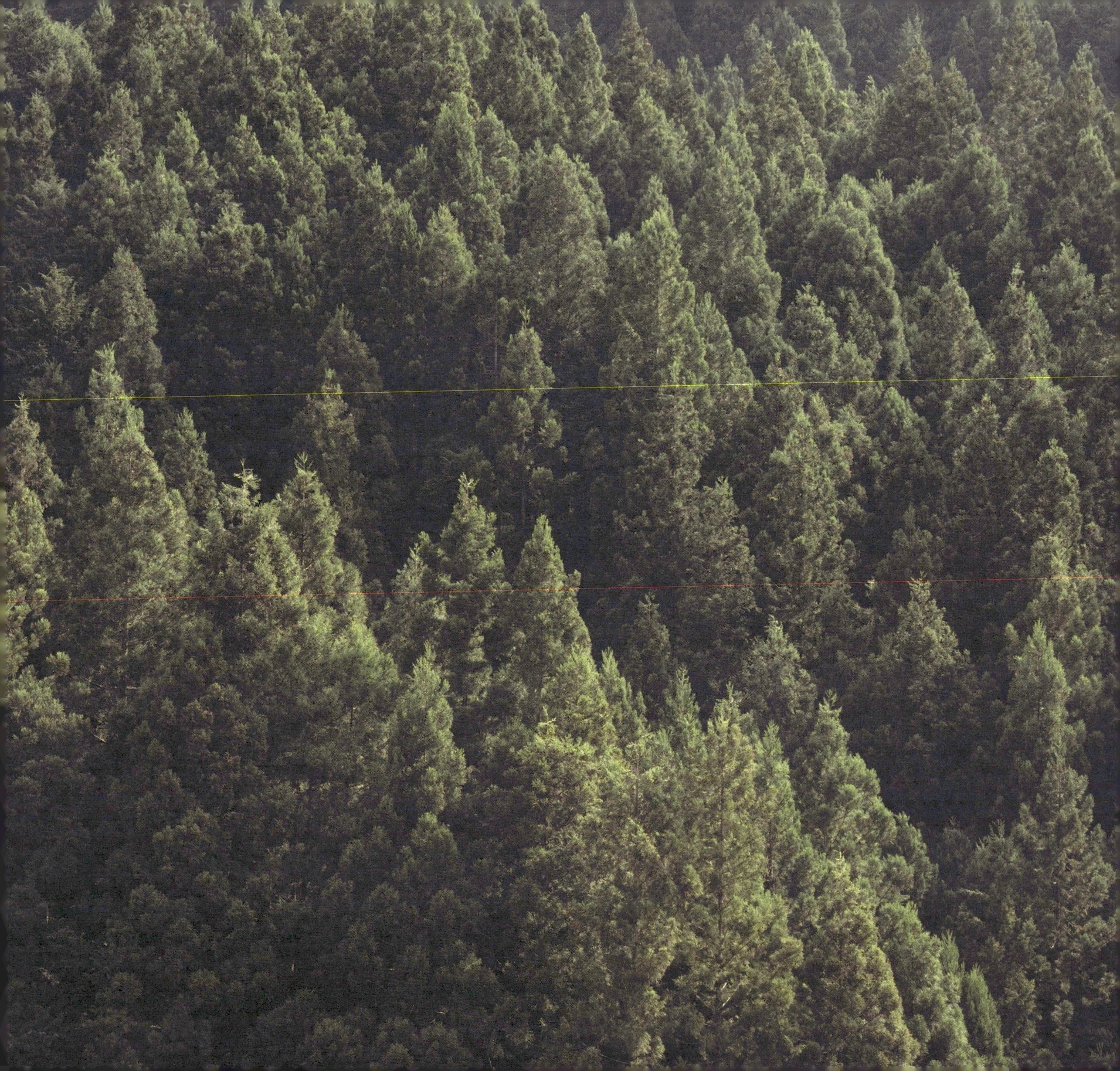

COMING TO MY SENSES

The largest city in the world, Tokyo, has given rise to a philosophy that pushes its practitioners to immerse themselves in the very environment it is not. A forest can offer a therapy that has gained traction around the world and can be a balm for urban life. My notions of nature are expanded as I use my senses to navigate the way of the forest.

TOKYO HUSTLE

The neon lights of Tokyo wrap around me like a blanket of colour as I spin in the center of Shibuya Crossing. A swarm of people engulfs me in the busiest intersection in the world. I feel dazed as I adjust to the scene. For the first time in my life, I am a stranger in this world—it's as though everything is a millisecond off, like watching a dubbed film where lips don't move in sync with sounds. It's unsettling but intriguing all at once.

Screens with animated characters flash, followed by fast-paced commercials that zoom and pop in a way that only Japanese ads can. There are a dizzying number of signs on building facades, each lit up and curated to lure consumers into their camera store, sushi bar, or nightclub. The intensity that is Tokyo—an organized pulse of bigger and brighter—would make Times Square jealous in its mastery of the senses. I wonder if I am up for the challenge as a month of flying and filming sips at my already drained battery. Already exhausted, this may be too much.

After growing up in Toronto and working my first real job in New York City, I am no stranger to large cities, but nothing can prepare you for being in the largest city in the world. Its futuristic synchronicity is something to marvel at. From an organized customs experience as we entered the country to a seamless cab ride to our hotel in one of the city centres, the metropolis feels utopian. Looking at the clean streets with steady traffic, bustling public transport, and courteous commuters, my preconceived notions of a megacity are challenged. My North American urban concepts want to superimpose themselves on my experience the way the outline of a lightbulb lingers if you gaze at its filament for too long.

After four weeks of long-haul travel and filming, my health and optimism are nearly worn out. Landmark after landmark, interview after interview, I am mentally drained. With the finish line in sight, my body begins to slow down to conserve its energy. I crave quiet and rest but am simultaneously amazed by the spectacle that is Tokyo. Japan is my eighth country in thirty-three days and, after thousands of kilometres and seven red-eye flights, my capacity to process is at a minimum. I am excited to explore the city, but the grey buildings and crowd seem like a daunting task to tackle.

I remind myself that I may not have this opportunity again. I think back to my junior high cross-country races and the advice I was once given by a coach: "It takes more energy to start and stop than to keep going." So, I take a deep breath and soak in my environment, rationing my focus as the scene competes for my attention.

As I stare at Tokyo's digital horizon, a new vision comes into focus. I see a strange dichotomy between the familiar and the foreign. Tokyo is enamoured with the West but is steadfast in its commitment to its culture. For instance, the omnipresent 7-Eleven stores look recognizable from the outside; however, inside, they break all conventions. Instead of stale ham and cheese sandwiches, I find shrimp-wrapped delicacies and octopus jerky. Rows of seaweed rice rolls with sour cherry centres or cream-filled pastries—even in mere convenience stores—showcase Japan's trait of elevating everything.

[previous page] The trees of Okutama
[opposite] The lights of Tokyo

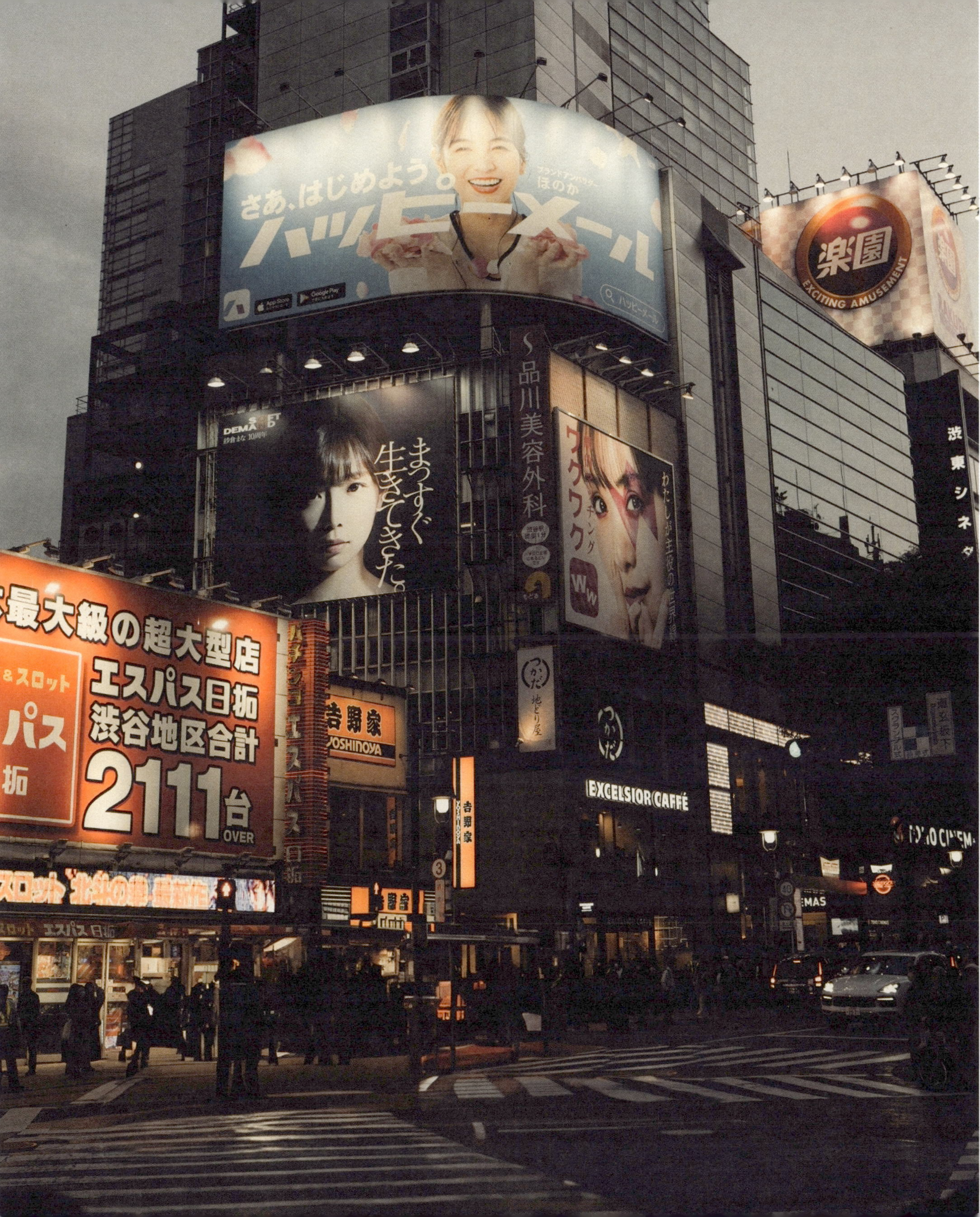

さあ、はじめよう。
ハッピーメール
楽園
EXCITING AMUSEMENT
まっすぐ生きてきた。
品川美容外科
ワクワク
最大級の超大型店
エスパス日拓
渋谷地区合計
2111台
OVER
吉野家
YOSHINOYA
EXCELSIOR CAFFÉ
スロット エスパス日拓

A DAY OF SURPRISES

I met Toshi, a local filmmaker, through his production company in Japan. When I introduce myself to him in the hotel lobby, his initial lack of excitement hints at a rather unenthusiastic day ahead. But, when our small crew comprising only James and Braeden appears, cameras in tow, Toshi's demeanour transforms. He had braced himself for a day plagued by the sluggishness of a large crew. Instead, he finds himself amidst an energetic guerrilla shooting spree. Ignited by the enthusiastic youth of our team members, we are off.

We start by visiting some typical landmarks, but his tourism route quickly changes as he relaxes into the role. A detour through local alleys and an indoor market spanning 200 metres of tiny restaurants and eateries is our first destination. We walk through the buzz of people eating and chefs searing dishes with steam rising from behind every counter. The wood interior contrasts with bold Japanese ink signage, and red drapes divide the countless diners. For the first time, I truly sense the tradition of Japan.

Emerging from this gastronomic tunnel, we enter the legendary neighbourhood of Harajuku. Famed for its eccentric fashion, Harajuku is an amalgamation of contemporary urban trends and traditional Japanese aesthetics. Bright Hello Kitty backpacks adorn storefronts, school-uniformed kids scamper about, and local artists showcase their craft.

Toshi signals for us to follow him into one art studio, a tiny second-floor space. Inside, shiny plastic, furry leggings, and cat ears dot the shelves. Two girls dressed in the fashion typical to Harajuku work the counter and graciously pose for my photo, each flashing peace signs with their heads tilted to the side and one leg lifted behind—a classic pose on cue, their pink and purple hair and neon leggings perfectly in sync.

As I leave the electrifying maze of Harajuku, a stark contrast awaits me. The calm expanse of the Meiji Jingu gardens sprawls out before my eyes. Entering the gardens, I step into a different era, worlds away from the relentless beat of Tokyo. It's as if the universe, sensing my need for peace, is guiding me from the clamour of the modern to the hushed whispers of the ancient, from the urban jungle to a pocket of natural tranquility.

The gardens are a sanctuary. I walk beneath a canopy of towering trees, their branches whispering reassurance as the breeze floats through the leaves. This sound resonates and comforts me, reminiscent of the giant poplar tree outside my childhood window. Its rustling, a familiar music, brings me back into the moment. The weight of the city's intensity begins to lift, replaced by a peaceful rhythm that resonates with every step I take on the gravel path. As I venture deeper, massive torii gates loom ahead, marking a sacred transition. Crafted from cypress wood and towering in height, these iconic Shinto gateways signal my entrance into a realm where reverence and serenity reign.

Places like this are what drew me to Tokyo. It's not the fast-paced urban setting I seek but the quiet of nature. Japan has given rise to a philosophy called shinrin-yoku, or forest bathing. Tomorrow, I'll meet with Dr. Kagawa—a researcher who will show me a setting even more dramatic than this. I am here to learn about how he was able to validate and measure the positive physiologic response to spending time in the natural world. His research has shown that in the forest our bodies are at peace: Our blood pressure drops, our minds forget their distractions, and we are saturated with natural chemicals from plants and trees called phytoncides, which improve our immune function. More than this, the air is clean, there is space to move, and the beneficial disorder of nature commands our attention and pulls us away from ruminating thoughts. I feel it, and I break free of my fatigued fog for a moment as clarity washes over me.

The shrine's grounds reveal more wonders to me now that I am alert. I come across walls adorned with decorative sake barrels, or kazaridaru. These barrels are art in themselves, wrapped in straw and showcasing intricate designs, representing offerings of rice wine to the enshrined deities. Their significance, bridging the shrine's spirituality with Japan's cultural traditions, stands out against the backdrop of the dense forest.

In the heart of the shrine, a scene of universal beauty unfolds before me. A traditional wedding procession gracefully weaves its way through the courtyard. The attendees, dressed in elegantly simple garments, maintain a comfortable pace. The bride, beautiful and serene, is shielded from the sun by a red umbrella, casting a warm glow over her and her groom. The buzz of the crowd stops, and a hush falls over us all in unison. A surreal feeling washes over me as I am immersed in the moment. The bustle of Tokyo now seems far, far away.

Visiting the Meiji Jingu gardens is a salve for my mind. Amidst a city that seems constantly moving, this sacred space provides me with a short but tranquil oasis for reflection. It's a needed reprieve from the constant stimulus of travel and gives me clarity and a more positive perspective. Again, I find myself drifting to the past, reminding me of my backyard, the solitude of the forest surrounding our home on Newfoundland's coast. The forest is a constant comfort in everyday life normally, its absence provides the opportunity for stress to take hold and grow. Little by little, flight by flight, I see how the pressures—even positive pressures—have accumulated without my normal relief and breath of time in nature. From steaming Delhi, to crowded airports, there has been a relentless tug at my mind. I am eagerly anticipating tomorrow's exploration of the forests of Okutama—the home of the therapy trail designed by Dr. Kagawa himself. I stare at the trees swaying in the breeze and notice them casting long shadows on the path before me. It reminds me of our final task for the day: to watch nature's final performance and witness the sun as it dips below Tokyo's skyline.

We return to Shibuya, having pinpointed an ideal spot in a tower for an unobstructed view of the horizon. The sun gracefully descends between the towering skyscrapers while giant video screens flash their movies and advertisements. Swarms of people move in orchestrated chaos, crossing the iconic X-shaped intersection as twilight deepens. Streetlights awaken, and lights flicker on in tall buildings, heralding the city's evening act. Mesmerized, I watch the sun's final moments, its image searing a renewed impression of Tokyo into my consciousness.

With the day's filming behind us, Toshi leads us through the bustling streets until we reach an unassuming building. We climb four flights of stairs to the entrance of a quaint, glass-fronted restaurant. Beyond the central area, the space opens up, revealing a sprawling local sushi eatery. Toshi takes the reins in ordering, and we toast our chilled beers. I savour every bite of my sashimi and miso soup. Retrieving my phone, I navigate to my "Favourites" folder and open "bucketlist.doc." I read down the list until I find what I'm looking for: Eat sushi in Tokyo. The cursor blinks with its patient rhythm before transforming into a checkmark. Pocketing my phone, I smile, content in this perfect moment.

I realize it was the infusion of nature that brought me across the finish line on this day. From an attitude of reluctant participation to one that achieves a goal in life, I credit my change in perspective to my reconnecting with nature. We should all remember that in life, there are tools all around us that we can employ to listen to and support our bodies and our minds. Nature may be one of the most powerful modalities we can use. I am excited to learn more about the science of forest therapy, but that's not until tomorrow. I sit back, intent on just enjoying today.

THE HEALING TRAILS OF OKUTAMA

The journey by train from Tokyo's buzzing Shinjuku Station to Okutama deconstructs the built environment before my eyes. With each passing minute, the imposing office towers dwindle, replaced by low houses, then stretches of open land, and finally, a horizon touched with green. The transformation from urban concrete to leafy nature offers a visual metaphor for the change in pace my mind needed.

Even the crowd metamorphoses before my eyes. Business suits and modern fashion gave way to backpacks and hiking boots. The mass of people, like the towering buildings we left behind, spread out and give me room to breathe. Before long, I have space and seats and quiet. I am seeking what others on the train already know—that the forests of Okutama are a remedy for the intensity of the big city and the urgency of urban life.

In Okutama, we're greeted by a local forest therapist, Akemi, a guide who will introduce me to the art and science of shinrin-yoku, or forest bathing. This isn't just a nature walk; it is therapy, a mindful immersion into the senses of nature. This practice has been adopted around the world, but it began here, in this forest.

Akemi is calm and kind. She is clearly committed and well studied for the adventure. She presents herself with a lively peacefulness. We begin with an offering at a Shinto temple at the top of the trail. The Shinto faith of Japan is deeply intertwined with nature, promoting the belief that forests, mountains, and rivers are sacred and inhabited by spirits.

Our offering is a way of showing respect and reverence to these spirits before visiting their home. As I drop my coins into the offering plate, they fall between the wooden dividers with a hollow rattle. It's not just the coins I release; I feel my stress begin to leave my body and my awareness return from this mindful moment.

We bow and make our way to the staircase beside the shrine. It leads to a small river that winds its way through the steep hills of lush trees. The rocky shoreline is made of countless eroded river rocks. Here, I have my first encounter with nature's patience, a seemingly timeless exercise to roll rocks to their balanced form. This is where Akemi tests my blood pressure and heart rate with expert agility. I know mine are higher than usual, which she confirms. The impact of the forest is measurable, and establishing a baseline before its treatment helps validate the shinrin-yoku approach. It also helps reinforce behaviour, even in the absence of the guide. I hope the program works for me as it does its patients.

A barefoot river walk is my opening order of therapy. The cold water numbs my tired feet, and the lapping current nudges me into embracing the feeling of this setting. I gingerly step through the stream as the hard stones massage my feet and the water gurgles around me. The smell of the clean, beer bottle-coloured water carries me to my childhood and our cabin by the Miramichi River. My family and I would spend all summer in that river, and now I find myself reflexively looking for tadpoles and minnows through the sheen of the water. At this moment, I am a child again. The memories feel so real; it's as though, brushed away, dormant and forgotten, they now float to the surface like the bubbles from the babbling brook.

"Pick a rock," Akemi instructs me as if reading my mind. Coming from a family of geologists, it has always been a tradition to take a stony souvenir from memorable stops. I find one, round and clean, that reminds me of the worry stone my father used to carry. I am unexpectedly bombarded with emotions and realize it has been too long since I have ventured into this corner of my mind. If this is the first task, what lies in store for the rest of the hike?

Rock in hand, I wade out of the water to the shore where Akemi is methodically stacking stones. "See how high you can make one," she instructs.

My competitive spirit ignited, I begin my audit of the beach for the flattest, most balanced rocks and stack them slowly, one on the other. The miniature tower teeters with each new stone. Concentrating on each pebble's shape, size, and weight focuses my mind, and I find the clutter of fatigue drifting away. I am playing with rocks on the shoreline like a child, and it puts me at peace. My nervous system powers down, and I'm quieted into the activity. Invested in this process, I try one more rock and knowingly smile as the tower topples. It's an Icarian attempt to go higher but with a positive reward. Looking up, Akemi acknowledges my effort. I check in with my body and can feel my heart beating more slowly and my breathing becoming deep and gentle. She smiles at my awareness and signals that it's time to move on.

We begin our walk up the trail of soft cedar chips that crack underfoot. The spongy softness fills my nostrils with a woodsy fragrance, but there's competition for my olfactory attention from the aromatic blend of blooming flowers and trees all around. The faint chirping of birdsong fills my ears. Every sense is heightened, every detail sharply invigorating me with a clarity that had seemed elusive in the city.

Okutama is a forest of towering evergreens. The park arborists remove their branches for the entire length of the trees, creating a canvas of linear trunks that challenge the mind in a visual puzzle. It is nature's cathedral. Here, I feel small, yet a part of something vast and intricate.

The moment that captures the essence of this therapy for me is my instruction on a bridge. Akemi asks me to stand still and to listen intently. There, amid the profound silence, I hear it—the soft trickle of a hidden waterfall, a sound I would've missed had I not focused on my senses. The creativity of the therapy resonates with a playful genius at this moment, and I realize how brilliant this approach is. The insights gained are immediate, and the mechanism is relatable and insightful. There is no more explicit way to demonstrate distraction than to unveil the world you have been missing by letting you pull the curtain of clutter aside for yourself.

I meander along the trails and watch the treetops sway in the wind. The path switches back and forth up the mountainside as the giant cedars reach skyward. Emerging near the top of the trail, Akemi motions for me to come and see a beautiful flowering bush.

"Use your 'insect eyes'," she instructs as I take in the colourful blossoms and delicate petals. Bright pink and perfect, they are a miracle of nature. "Now use your 'eagle eyes' and look up," she says as she motions to the horizon. My vision shifts as I focus on the sky. The expertly planned trail is cut away to reveal a panoramic view of the valley. Tall mountains decorate the distance as hills and treetops add their dark emerald colour to the picture. The contrast is moving, and the impact of this sensual trickery makes me smile. Got me again, I think as I marvel at the scene.

Gazing at the perfect picture, I see a small trail of smoke rising from the woods, signalling our next stop in the valley. A small wooden structure overhangs a ravine, glowing a soft, warm hue. It looks cozy and inviting in the cool spring air.

I approach the rest station and peer through its window as I open the door. Walking in, I am greeted by Dr. Kagawa, the founder of forest therapy; his entrance is timed perfectly to coincide with my first-hand immersion on the trail. He carries himself with a serene calmness. He speaks softly and intentionally, never wasting words or over-expressing an idea. He delivers his insights and knowledge with humble confidence, smiling after conveying words of wisdom.

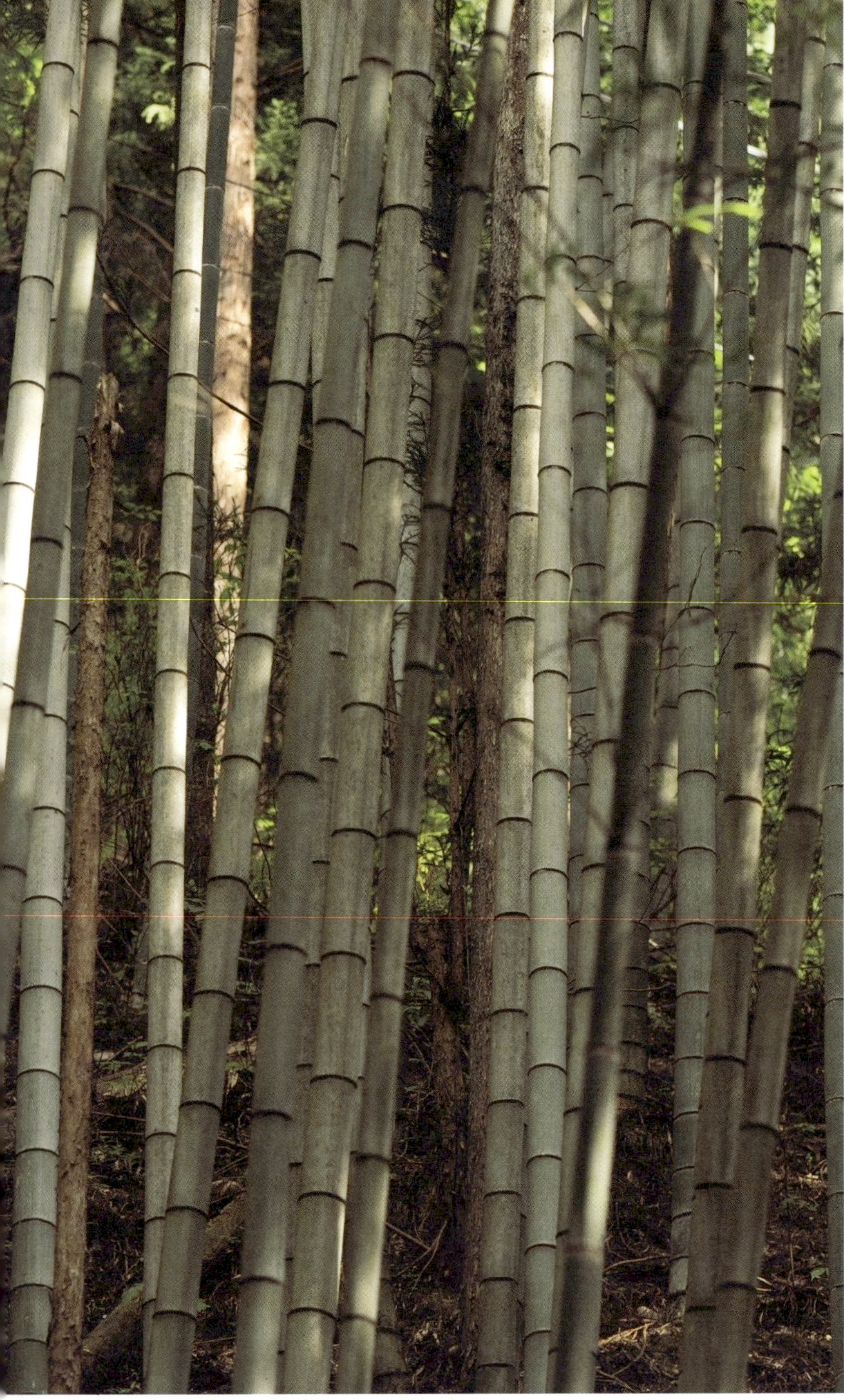

His mannerisms are relaxed—like the trees that sway gently in the mountain breeze. He blends with his environment, and I am instantly comfortable.

Forest bathing is an inclusive therapy that helps patients connect with the natural world while addressing physical and mental health challenges. These formal therapeutic moments seamlessly blend with the environment and tap into awareness triggered by the forest experience. This helps speed up counselling by priming the patient to be present, aware, and disconnected from their day-to-day stressors.

I see steam rising from a teapot and smell fresh gingerbread cookies on the table. There are large glass panoramic windows looking over the gorge, its breathtaking view chosen for obvious reasons. A small wood fire burns in the corner, and the orange and yellow flames flick at the stove's window, reminding me of my shed back home. Akemi and I remove our shoes and don slippers, a familiar Japanese ritual. She takes me to a small room with a glass window to the right of the central area. The room is like a miniature auditorium with padded benches staggered on different levels before the window. She asks me to lie down and close my eyes. I lay on the surprisingly comfortable bench as she hits a chime.

"In the last thirty days, think of one thing you are grateful for," she says, followed by, "today, think of something you saw that was beautiful."

The questions then change to those of greater introspection: "What could you have done better this week?" and "What are you most proud of?" This exercise, a stoic evaluation, capitalizes on the mindfulness stimulated by nature to interpret our day-to-day unconscious.

Following the meditation, we sip hibiscus tea by the fire, accompanied by the warm cookies. The herbal tea and tart gingerbread stir my previously neglected sense of taste. The fire crackles and pops as I recount my curated selection of birch and spruce firewood back home with pride.

Warm and content, we depart the cabin to visit our final therapy station. Emerging into a clearing, we see metal wire benches that have been artistically shaped to lie down upon to watch the clouds drift by. The curious design elevates my legs to commit me fully to the relaxing endeavour. Staring at the clouds drifting by, I realize fragrant bushes surround me. My mind drifts and quizzes itself . . . I'd like to know how many obscure sensory details I've missed on my countless hikes along the East Coast Trail of Newfoundland.

Often, amid our busy lives, we're in nature, but not with nature. We see, but we don't observe; we hear but don't listen.

Now, eyes opened, ears tuned, and taste and smell alive, we walk toward the trail exit. Dr. Kagawa walks quietly behind Akemi and me, his presence calm and relaxed. He observes silently, embodying the calm and focus that forest therapy promotes. His slow, intentional words, interspersed with pauses, allow the forest sounds to create dimension between his thoughts and add a new layer to our experience.

Dr. Kagawa continues to elaborate on one of his most fascinating discoveries. He has shown that shinrin-yoku can reduce our stress hormones. These are the hormones that cloud our minds, increase our anxiety, and make our hearts race. Being in the forest pauses the stimulus that causes these hormones to be released, evoked by thoughts of meetings, calls, and deadlines. Dr. Kagawa has shown that a dose of nature has a greater impact on improving our health than many medications physicians dispense without hesitation. Somehow, humans now find it easier to take synthetic drugs than to immerse ourselves in the natural world. This is why Dr. Kagawa calls his form of therapy "forest bathing"; he believes it should be a daily ritual that cleanses our bodies and minds from the artificial world we lather ourselves in.

Sauntering down the path, I am in no hurry. I find myself running my hand along the trees' bark as I pass and listening to the wind in the leaves. I smell the dampness of the moss that lines the trail and see water drops trickle from the rocky ledges. I'll be able to revisit this memory, adding to my collection of diamonds and waiting to be triggered the next time I am present in nature.

As the forest walk concludes, the tangible health benefits of forest therapy become evident in my body. The serene environment and the mindful practices embedded in our journey have orchestrated a noticeable drop in my blood pressure. This change manifests as a sense of deep tranquility and lightness. My breathing, now calmer and more rhythmic, mirrors the gentle pace of the forest itself, and my heart rate has slowed, aligning with nature's peaceful, unhurried rhythm. Mentally, there's a newfound quietude; my mind, often cluttered with the constant buzz of thoughts, now feels clearer and more focused. This mental stillness allows for a richer, more reflective sense of the world around me. I'm acutely aware of the symphony of natural sounds, the intricate patterns of the leaves, and the subtle play of light through the tree canopy. This heightened sensory awareness, coupled with physiological changes, encapsulates the value of forest therapy. It's not just a walk in the woods—it's a transformative experience that rejuvenates the body, calms the mind, and enriches the soul, leaving me with a sense of well-being and connection to the natural world.

Okutama was more than just a day away from Tokyo's hustle, it was a reminder—to pause, to feel, to be. We can find our little forest to bathe in, even surrounded by skyscrapers, neon lights, televisions, and cell phones. Forest therapy is a blend of purposeful silence and mindful observation. It peels back the layers of sensory overload that often shroud our perception, revealing the vibrant senses of life that thrive beneath. Okutama's trails have imprinted a profound truth: that the antidote to our modern ailments does not lie in the complex fabrications of human design but in the simple, elemental connection we share with the natural world.

So, whether it's a quiet park corner or a potted plant in your office, take time to create rituals in nature. Stop thinking and instead engage all your senses in your surroundings—herbal tea and gingerbread cookies are highly recommended.

[opposite] Visual trickery of the trail

TAKE A FOREST BATH

BEGIN WITH MINDFULNESS: Start your forest therapy with a quiet moment to centre your thoughts. Commit to leaving your worries behind and opening your senses to the experience.

EXPLORE THE VISUAL TAPESTRY: Look for patterns in how vines climb, or shadows play on the forest floor. Notice all the different greens and how the sunlight flickers through the leaves. Spot the contrast between the rugged bark and delicate ferns.

DISCOVER NATURE'S BOUQUET: Seek out new scents by gently brushing your hands against leaves and flowers, releasing their unique fragrances. Take a deep breath and smell the earth and the plants.

INDULGE IN TEXTURE: Touch the objects in your environment; feel how the tree bark is bumpy and the rocks are cool. Take off your shoes and feel the varied textures of the earth beneath your feet, from soft moss to the solidity of rocks.

ABSORB THE QUIETUDE: Close your eyes and identify subtle sounds you might otherwise miss—the distant trickle of a stream or the soft flutter of butterfly wings, the rustle of leaves or the small sounds of animals moving around.

SAVOUR NATURAL FLAVOURS: Pack a small snack like nuts or apple slices to enjoy a simple, clean taste that complements your natural surroundings.

OUR FOREST THERAPISTS

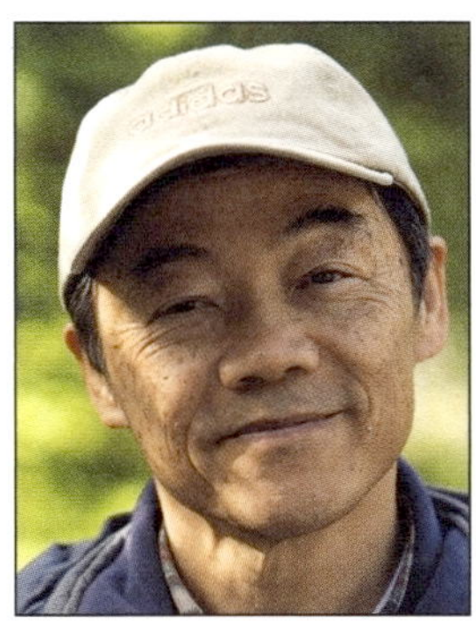

DR. KAGAWA—FOUNDER OF FOREST THERAPY: Quietly convincing, Dr. Kagawa has quantified the value of spending time in nature for our health. He coined the term "forest therapy" and has published over seventy-five papers on the topic. His work has guided forest therapy practices globally, and his recipe for the creation of accessible trails is the blueprint on which other progressive programs base their work. By stimulating the five senses, forest therapy combines traditional therapy and guided meditation to create experiential, psychological healing.

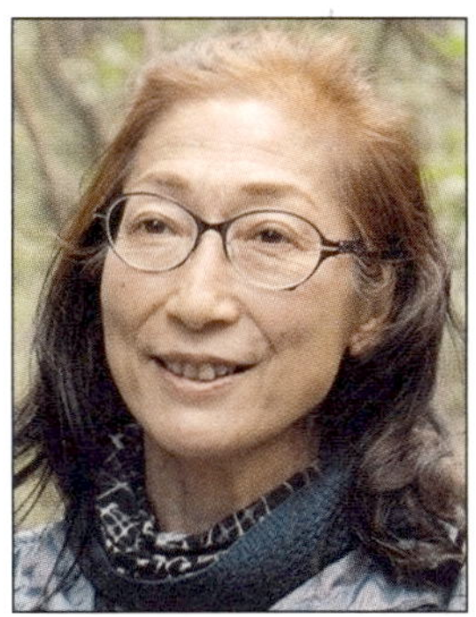

AKEMI—FOREST GUIDE: Akemi is a certified forest therapy guide and practitioner. Studying under Dr. Kagawa and running programs on the healing trail of Okutama, Akemi draws out subtle, thoughtful additions to the therapeutic process. From stacking stones to feeling textured tree barks, Akemi seeks to inspire and teach so that when you leave the trails of Okutama and wander your own forests, her lessons follow—whatever route you choose.

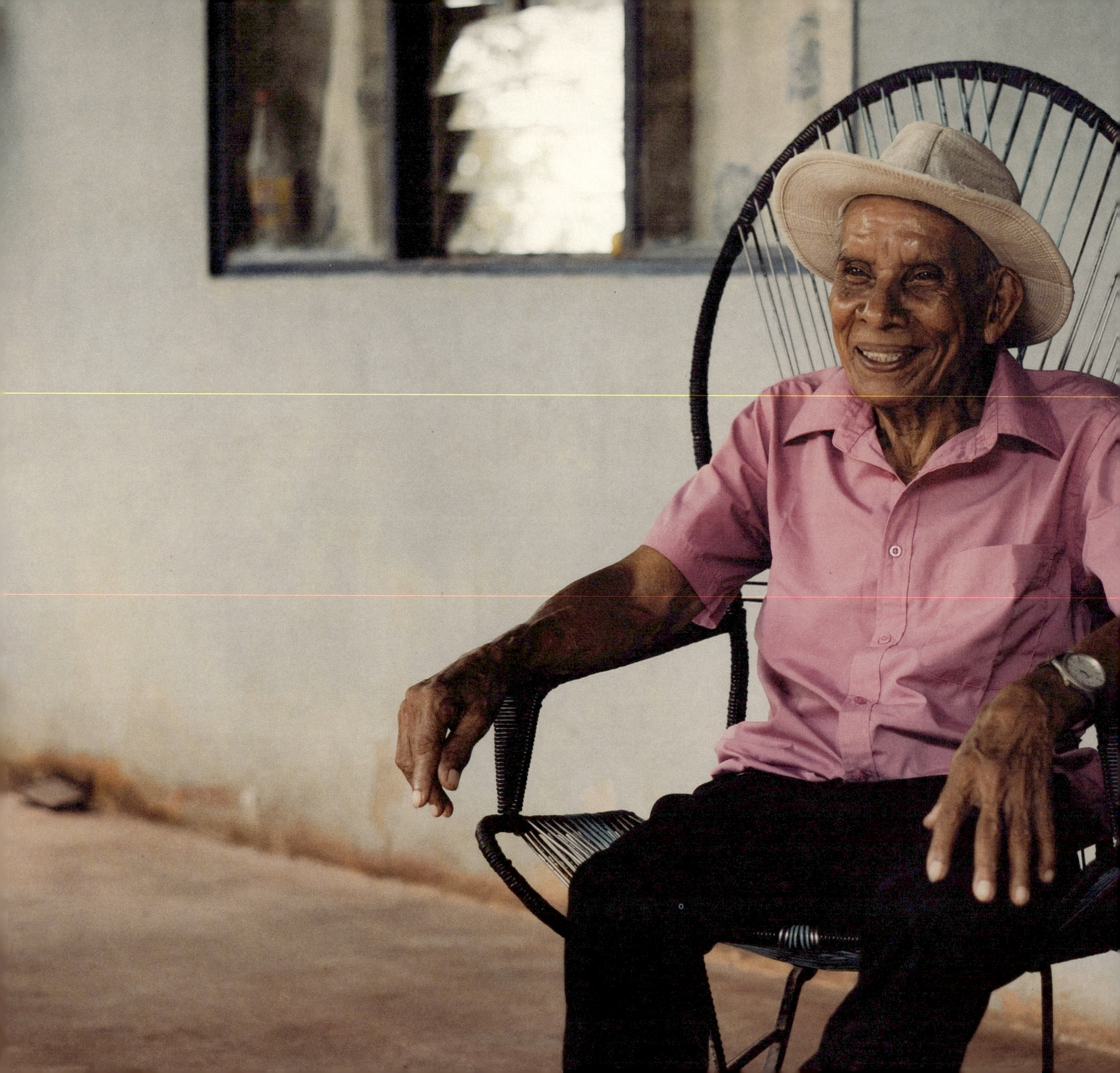

PURE LIFE

Down the dusty roads of Costa Rica hides a pocket of longevity where seniors are cherished. Cradled in community and tradition with a hearty helping of purpose and simplicity, centenarians evade loneliness to live long, full lives.

PURA VIDA

"This is the spot," announces our guide as he gestures toward a humble wooden home nestled off the dirt road. Around the yard, roosters and chickens wander freely while a lazy dog basks in the morning sun. Smoke slowly drifts from a covered area to the left of the house, mixing with the morning haze of the rainforest.

As we approach, several family members greet us with open arms. Their warmth is immediate and enveloping, making us feel instantly welcome. They offer me a mug of coffee, a gesture particularly appreciated at this early hour. I can tell immediately it will be good; Costa Rica has a reputation for its exceptional java. Settling down at a picnic table, I take in my surroundings. The kitchen at the back of the home is alive with activity—red-hot coals consume the small logs fed into the wood-fired stove. A humble assortment of pots and pans hangs on the wall, and ingredients are thoughtfully arranged and ready for my visit.

Here, I have the pleasure of meeting Donna Maria, a centenarian deeply connected to her family and the tradition of cooking. At 101 years old, she embodies vitality, a living testament to the Costa Rican way of life, called Pura Vida, that values community, family, and simplicity.

When she emerges from her house, we exchange handshakes and greetings. Her hair is grey, and she is wearing a bright sundress for the occasion. Her eyes are large and searching, aware and vibrant for her age.

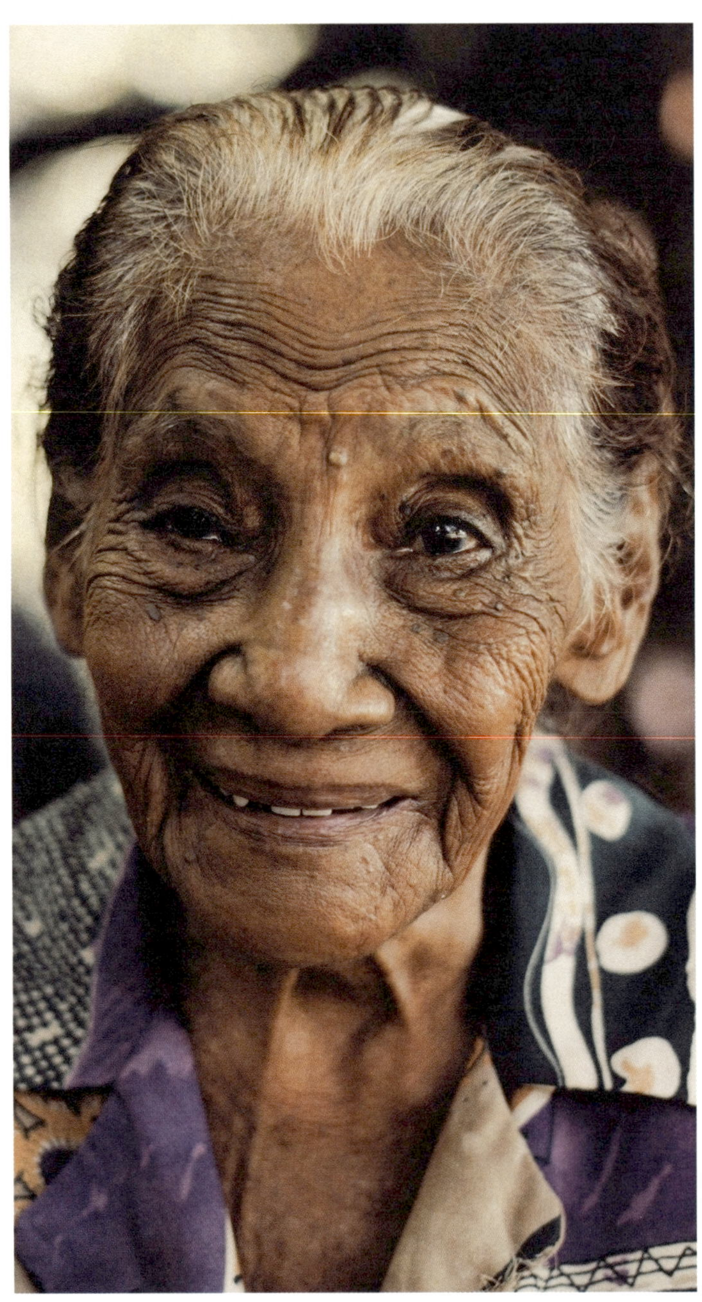

[previous page] Juan embracing Pura Vida
[above] Maria the chef; [opposite] Maria's humble home

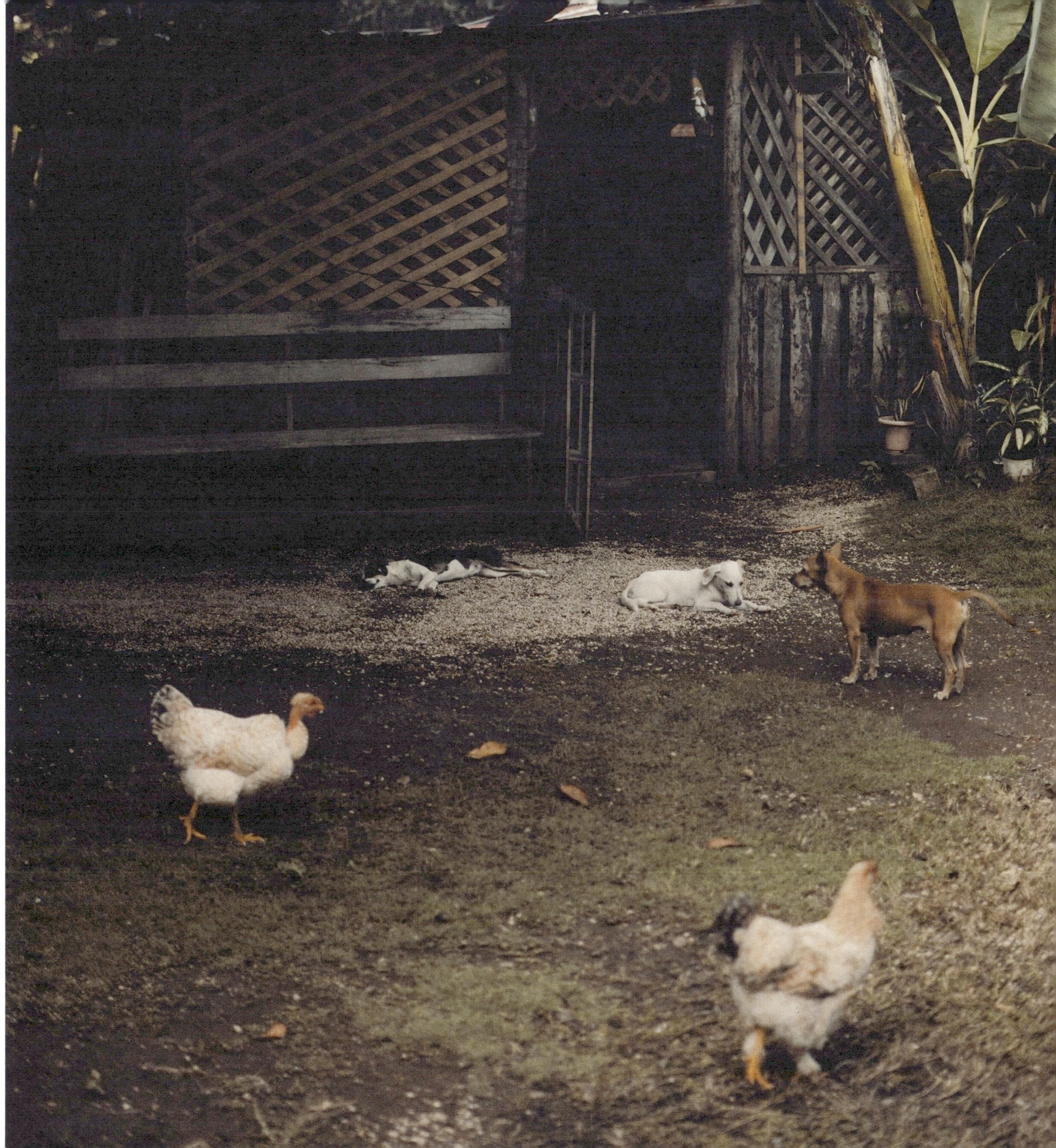

Without delay, Donna Maria gets down to business. She heads toward the back of the kitchen, signalling for me to follow. Although she stands no more than four and a half feet tall and moves slowly, she has an air of independence and authority. She has been cooking her entire life and has agreed to show me one of her favourite recipes.

We take our positions around the fire, relishing the thick aroma of wood smoke. Skillfully, she places a large, round pan over the stove, her experienced hands deftly positioning the coals with a small stick. Today, she will teach me how to make gallo pinto, a traditional Costa Rican dish. Her kitchen, though modest, has an aura of warmth and love; it's masterfully simple and holds decades of stories.

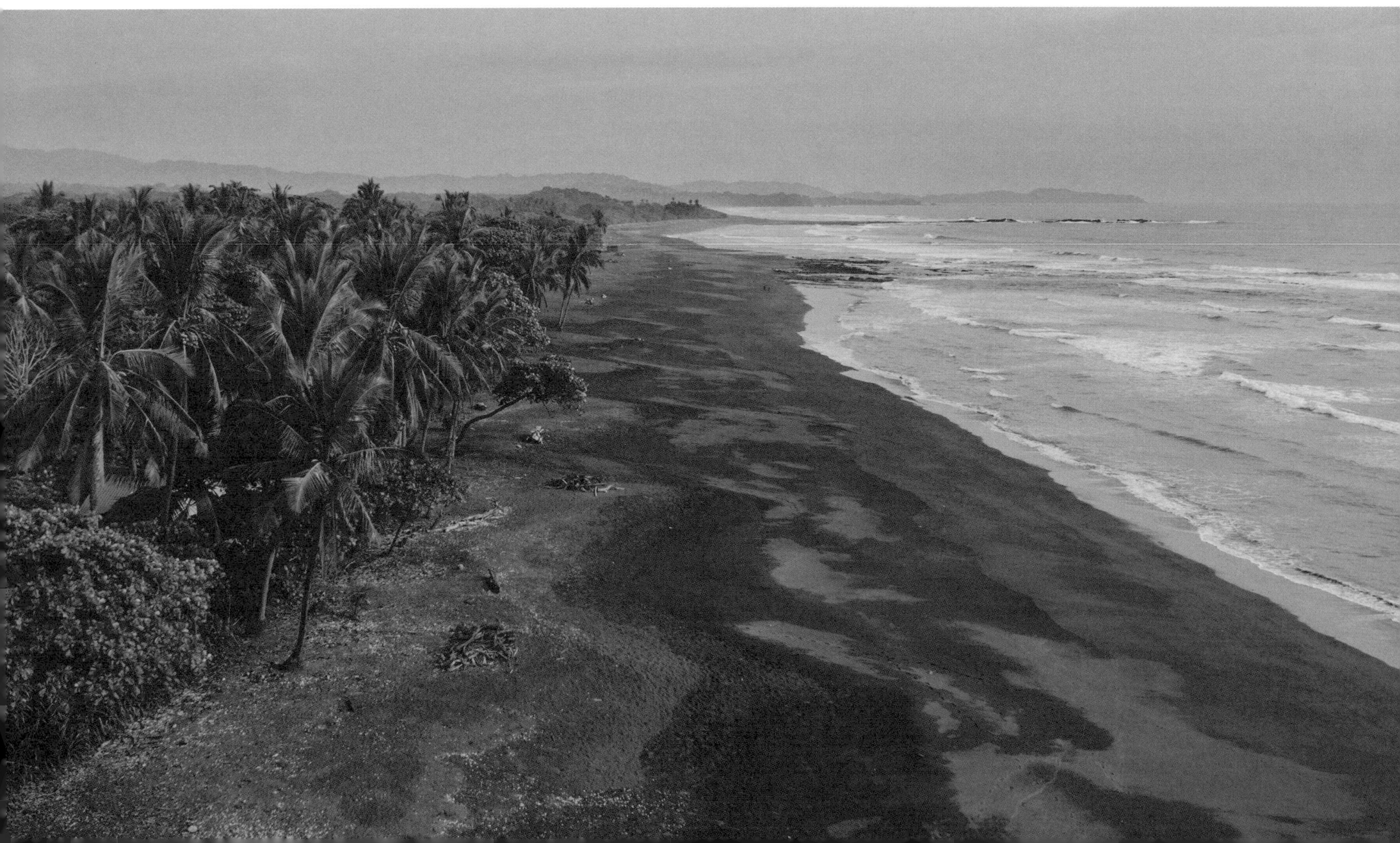

Her family, spanning four generations, from her daughter and granddaughter to the youngest, an energetic toddler, are all present, interpreting, explaining, and helping Donna Maria. There is a buzz of life all around. I feel so far removed from my home kitchen's organized and sterile subway-tiled convenience.

Donna Maria's instructions are concise yet meticulous. She begins with a drizzle of oil in the pan, then adds beans and a blend of aromatic spices. She calls out for ingredients to her seventy-something-year-old daughters, who quickly pass her the requested constituents. As we mix, she introduces rice and adds a uniquely Costa Rican flare: Lizano sauce. This cooking ritual, passed down through generations, transcends mere culinary preparation. It's a celebration of heritage, a means to nourish her family and soul. She has done this her entire life and still insists on it to this day—it is her own beautiful way to strengthen the connection with her family.

Her home is humble and unassuming but is a haven of love and togetherness. Here, in this simplest of places, wealth is measured not in material possessions but in the richness of relationships and the joy of shared experiences.

In North America, longevity is often pursued through medical advancements and material comfort. Yet, in contrast to Donna Maria's life, our quest for more years seems to have lost sight of what truly matters—living. As I observe Donna Maria surrounded by her loving family, I can't help but reflect on the stark contrast with our own approach to aging. In our society, older people are often seen as burdens and relegated to nursing homes, their wisdom and experience undervalued. The pandemic laid bare the profound impact of loneliness and isolation on our health, revealing a crisis of connection that lies in stark contrast to the close-knit communities of Costa Rica.

The concept has intrigued me for years, spurring a radio interview with Drs. Richard Schwartz and Jacqueline Olds from Harvard, authors of *The Lonely American*, who highlighted some startling statistics. Loneliness is not just a social issue but a health hazard and increases the risk of premature death by up to twenty-six per cent. Being alone is as bad for our health as obesity and smoking. Moreover, socially isolated individuals have a fifty per cent higher risk of developing dementia, a twenty-nine per cent higher risk of heart disease, and a thirty-two per cent higher risk of stroke.

I admire Donna Maria as she navigates her kitchen. She stops me from stirring as the beans and rice, a staple of the region's longevity foods, are finished. The hearty concoction wafts a sweet and savoury smell through the kitchen. I feel my stomach growl in anticipation, an inadvertent compliment to the chef. We serve our breakfast and sit at the table, where with the help of her oldest daughter, I get a chance to learn from Donna Maria.

She explains that in Costa Rica, family and community are the foundation on which society is built. Her community is the most important thing to her, but it triggers a pain that usually stays buried. She tears up as she ponders why she is still left here in this world, outlasting her siblings and several of her children. She admits to living a good life and wonders if she will ever leave this world, scared by the prospect of immortality. I see that longevity is both a blessing and a burden as losing those you love scars the heart.

Donna Maria turns to faith to help her process these questions and her circumstances—it provides her peace and a means to reflect on a well-lived life. Despite the inevitable losses that come with age, Maria's life is buffered by the constant presence and support of her loved ones. Her days are filled with purpose and connection, starkly contrasting with the isolation experienced by many in the rest of the Western world.

Longevity is not just about the length of our years but the depth of our connections. In the bustling cities and lonely suburbs, it's time we re-evaluate our priorities and redefine what it means to live a long, fulfilling life. As Donna Maria and her family show me, the secret to longevity might lie in the simple, timeless joys of community, family, and a good cup of coffee.

[opposite] The black sand of Ostinal beach on the Nicoya Peninsula

AMIGO AND ADVOCATE

Before we leave, our guide, Jorge, snaps a photo of me and the crew, along with Donna Maria and her family for his collection of stories.

Jorge, the head of the Blue Zones Association of Costa Rica, is intertwined with the more than 100 centenarians in the area. Charming and friendly, he interacts easily with his often hard-of-hearing, visually impaired, and mobility-challenged seniors. Each time we meet a new centenarian, they are overjoyed with his arrival, as are their families. This afternoon, we are invited to a 100-year-old's birthday party, and it's our job to get the cake. It might seem strange that someone from outside the family would have such an essential role in the party—until you learn more about Jorge's part in the community.

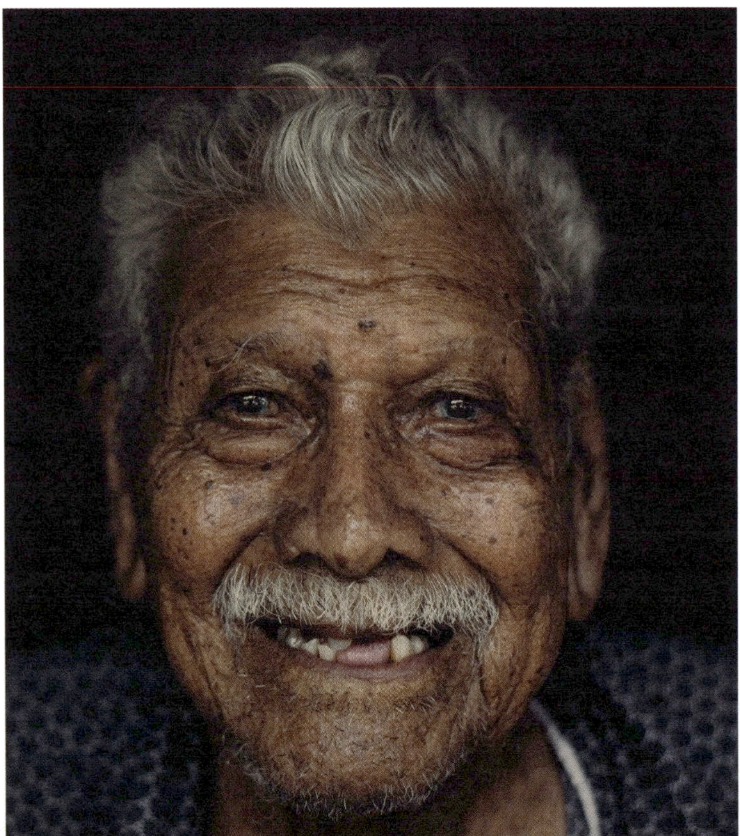

Over thirty years ago, he began researching seniors in the Nicoya area. Before urbanization and development, Costa Rican officials noticed a peculiar population emerging from the region. Nicoya, the small, dry tropical forest of the northwestern part of Costa Rica, is home to many long-lived individuals. It wasn't due to wealth, nor the medical system. They didn't have magic foods; instead, they ate some of the simplest foods imaginable. It was something else, perhaps the Pura Vida—or pure life—philosophy the area has coined, the social traditions, the climate, or the lack of crop pesticides. No one knew, so a young Jorge began interviewing all the senior citizens in the region. He did this yearly and watched many seniors age through their eighties, nineties, and past the century mark. Now older and wiser, he has had decades-long relationships with those he works with, and his association raises money for those vulnerable centenarians in a place where government pensions and RRSPs are a rare security for seniors.

With cake in hand, we arrive at the celebration, which is being held in the yard, with tents set up for shelter. Jorge is greeted like a hero. He is a champion for the elderly, and I think he is the kind of person we need to celebrate more in our community.

The party is a hive of activity with hundreds of guests. The entertainment, comprising Mantudos, or clowns, and a brass band entered just before us. These masked characters are the best babysitters for socializing parents, including

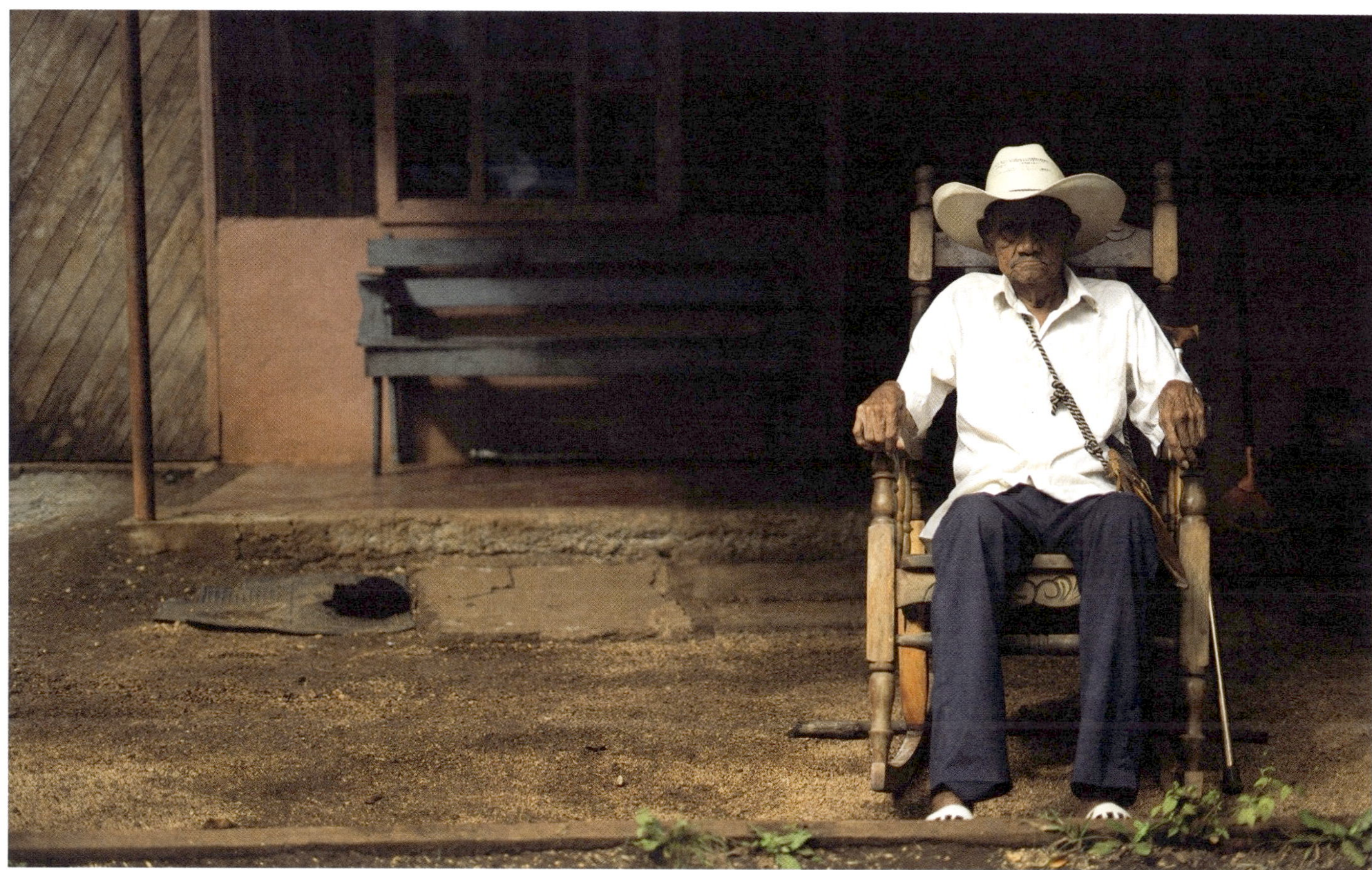

two demon-like dancers and a large bull. As the music plays, the children dart toward the monsters and tag them, only to be chased by the bull or the oversized demon, to their terrified delight.

We are here to honour the guest of the day. Yet amidst the celebration, the centenarian, another woman named Donna Maria, seems to gently drift between wakefulness and sleep, a quiet presence at her lively party. It is a poignant reminder of the gentle balance between celebrating life and honouring its natural progression.

Jorge, ever the gracious ambassador, takes the stage to welcome everyone and address the 100-year-old woman. As he presents the cake to her family, I stand to the side, observing this beautiful community tradition unfolding. The band then starts to play, their music weaving through the crowd and under the tents, where people huddle together, seeking shelter from the light rain.

The feast that follows is traditional, with rice wrapped in giant leaves being passed around. The Mantudos, now joined by the band, dance with an energy that rivals that of the children, who still pursue them with trepidation and excitement, their laughter filling the air.

As I absorb the scene, the party demonstrates the role of community and generations in gatherings. Food and drinks for the talkative types, music for the dancers, and games for the kids seamlessly intertwined into the gathering. We spend the day with partygoers and retire to our hotel after their celebration of fun, festivities, and longevity.

[opposite] 102-year-old veteran
[above] David the 101-year-old Bull Rider

THE SABANERO

The next day begins early. I am going to meet Ramiro, who, at 102 years old, stands as a living testament to the wonders of healthy aging. He is not just fit; he is the benchmark of vitality, often regarded as one of the fittest individuals in the world for his age. I have come here to understand how he has been able to achieve this feat but to do that, I have to get up before the sun.

As I approach, Ramiro sits in an old rocking chair overlooking his cows grazing in the field while his son-in-law does the milking—an activity Ramiro has regrettably assigned to others at this stage in his life. He greets me with a firm handshake and a big grin. He is small but strong and has a flicker of mischief in his eyes—his spirit undimmed by the passage of time. He has been active all his life, starting work in his early teens. This lifelong engagement in daily physical tasks contributes to his remarkable fitness and keeps him socially and mentally engaged.

"What's your secret?" I blurt out almost immediately, shocked by the vitality he exudes. Without hesitation, he tells me he is focused on having a purpose each day. This gets him up before the sun and gives his life meaning.

Adorned in a white stetson hat, pale red shirt, tan jeans, and cowboy boots, his attire speaks volumes of his identity as a proud Guanacaste sabanero. His distinctive style is matched only by his unique mannerisms, including his signature high-pitched chirps, a cultural hallmark of the Guanacastecos. This strong sense of identity significantly mitigates feelings of isolation and loneliness.

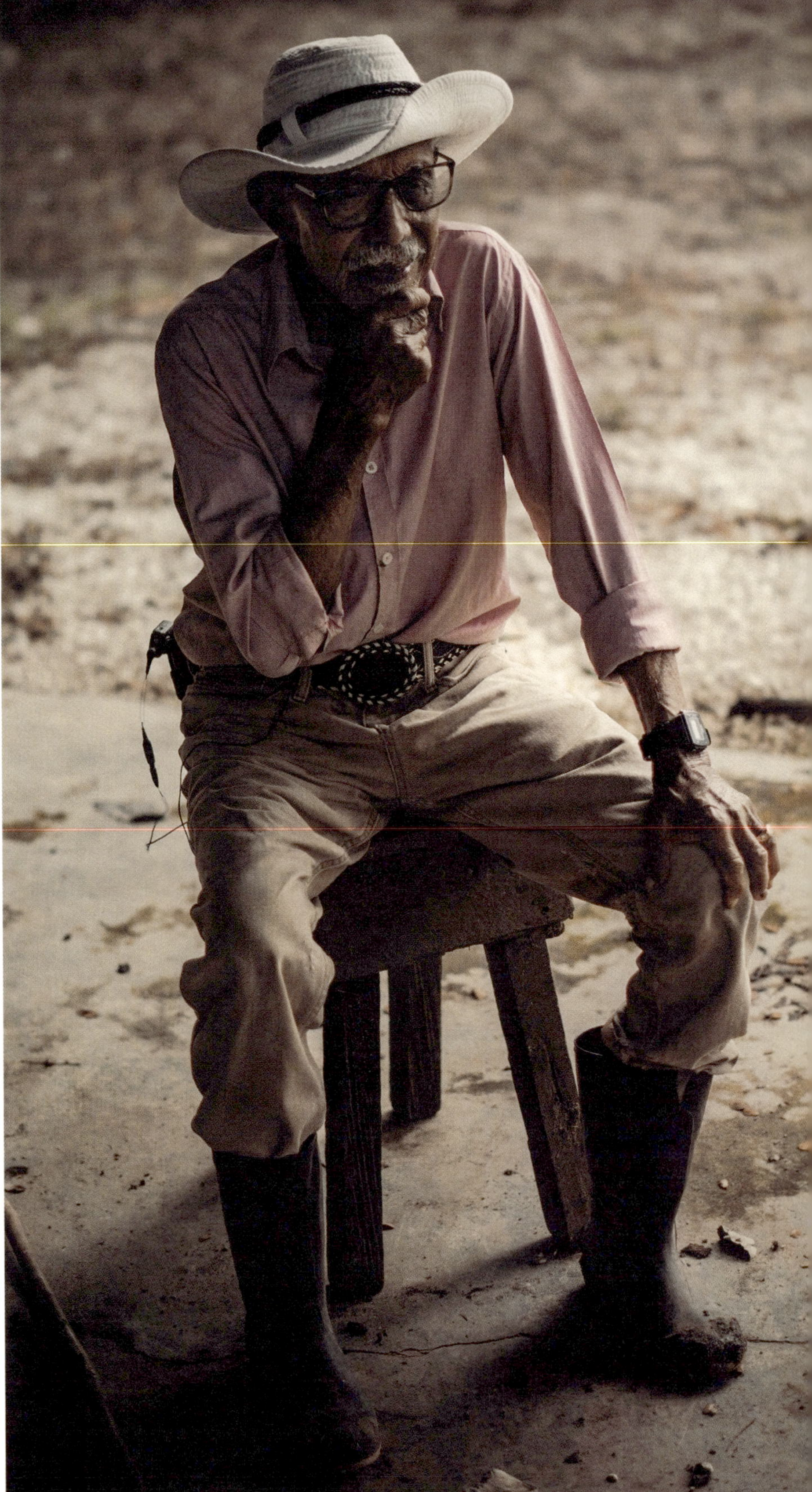

His days are filled with horseback riding, tending to his cows, and even dancing with friends. These activities provide vital social interaction, a cornerstone in maintaining mental health and emotional well-being in old age. Loneliness, often a silent epidemic among older people, is notably absent in Ramiro's life, replaced by a healthy network of family, friends, and community members.

With a neatly manicured grey mustache and glasses, Ramiro's face has graced the covers of magazines and documentaries. As we chat, he prepares to drive his herd with an agility that hides his years, swiftly mounting his horse in a fluid, effortless motion. He trots down the road, directing his cattle with a whistle and an ease that astonishes me. Watching him work, one might forget his centenarian status, for he moves better than many people half his age.

The cattle obediently follow his lead, turning up a trail toward the pasture. His control over these animals is a sight to behold. The cows move down the road in sync, turn a bend to a smaller dirt road, and then veer into a pasture. This is the daily routine each and every day of his life. He sees work not only as a means of income but as a tonic for aging and as necessary as oxygen. He shakes his head at his son-in-law, who doesn't share his enthusiasm and says, "He never milks the cows right." I chuckle because it's surprising to see someone so passionate about their work at this stage in life, especially when my own society rushes to retired stagnancy as soon as possible, with little contemplation on finding purpose during the next phase of life.

Once the task is complete, Ramiro turns to me and declares, with a straightforwardness born of a life lived in earnest, "It's time for breakfast." He jumps on his horse, and he is gone. Ramiro is a man of routines, so Jorge and I meet him back at his home. It's a simple dwelling that resonates with the warmth of family and history; his daughter transforms the fresh milk her husband collected into cheese while Ramiro's great-grandson nestles comfortably in his lap under a large tree in the backyard.

With a life as colourful as his, it is not surprising that his home is a veritable museum, its walls adorned with newspaper articles and photographs chronicling a century of stories. These mementos serve as a constant reminder of his valued place in the family and society, reinforcing his sense of self-worth and belonging.

The breakfast table is a familial affair, with Ramiro enjoying a hearty meal of gallo pinto and eggs. This intergenerational interaction, a daily occurrence in Ramiro's life, is crucial in maintaining his emotional health. He is still the breadwinner in the family, and his family demonstrates a weighty level of respect for his contribution. I learned that they have been incredibly successful with their ranch. Despite the humble environment, Ramiro and his family have created an enterprise that will support future generations. This legacy, this Pura Vida, is instilled within Ramiro's very being.

In Ramiro, we see the embodiment of inspiration. His daily life, steeped in physical activity, family connections, and a deep-rooted sense of purpose, offers a blueprint for aging with grace and vitality. His firm handshake as we part ways is not just a farewell but a testament to a life continually in motion. For Ramiro, every day is an opportunity for engagement, nurturing family ties, and another chance for meaningful work.

His story challenges our conventional notions of aging. In a world where the elderly are often sidelined, Ramiro stands as the model of what it means to age not just with longevity but with a contagious zest for life. He reminds us that age is but a number and that vitality, purpose, and connection are the true markers of a life well lived. His life is a powerful illustration of how maintaining strong social ties, engaging in regular physical activity, and having a sense of purpose can not only enhance the quality of life in the elderly but also provide a formidable shield against the loneliness that can otherwise diminish their golden years.

[opposite] Ramiro contemplating his story

A REMEDY FOR LONELINESS

As I travel deeper into the heart of Costa Rica's Blue Zone, I find myself reflecting on my own life. The experiences here, especially with these remarkable centenarians, have opened my eyes to different ways of life and kindled a newfound appreciation for my journey to finding companionship.

I find myself drifting to this thought as we bounce down pot hole-filled dirt roads to a hidden gem on the coast. It's the tiny town of Nosara and a place I know well. Perhaps the magic that instills longevity in this region has also intoxicated me, as I have been to this place six times before. I am typically not a repeat traveller, but the community's peace has always drawn me back. It's getting late, so I make my way to the water.

I find a comfortable spot to watch the day conclude and survey the beach. The waves are good today, and silhouettes of surfers put on a show for sunset seekers as dogs play on the beach. My wife and I visited this spot just last year. As the beauty of the scene unfolds, I'd normally reach over and hold her hand. I miss her acutely in this moment.

Our love story began later in life. I met Leanne through a chance encounter with friends, and from the outset, it was as if all the scattered pieces of my life had suddenly aligned. We fell in love instantly, and within a year, we were engaged and making life plans. Our wedding, held on the second anniversary of our first date, was intentional and beautifully simple. We were married by our best friend and wrote our own vows. Trying to express what I truly felt was like separating the colours in a beam of sunlight, an impossible puzzle where my heart's true feelings remained beyond the grasp of words.

We often joke about our "proximity infatuation," and just being near each other is enough to create peace in our lives. This deep-seated connection, a fusion of our souls, has guided me to explore new horizons, pursue my passions, and strive to be a better person. It's a bond that transcends the physical; it's a meeting of minds and hearts that has enriched every aspect of my life.

While inspiring and enlightening, my current journey in Costa Rica has also stirred a deep longing within me. As I film and document the lives of those who have found happiness in the warmth of their community and family, I find myself missing my own. There's an irony in my situation—while I am out here exploring the essence of communal joy and longevity, my heart aches for the familiar comfort of my own community in Newfoundland.

In St. John's, much like in the Blue Zone of Nicoya, there's a shared sense of familiarity and belonging that's hard to find elsewhere. Everyone knows each other, creating a comforting and empowering sense of trust. This strong sense of connection, I realize, is what I miss the most—it's the feeling of being a part of something larger than yourself, a feeling that resonates deeply with the ethos I've witnessed in Costa Rica.

Our well-being is intrinsically linked to our connections with others. When we find places where community is valued, we also find a buffer against loneliness. Those closest to us provide a network of support, companionship, and a sense of belonging—a powerful antidote to the isolation and alienation that often accompany modern life. Our descent from familial living and small tribes may be a de-evolution for our well-being. In a world where individualism is often celebrated, tight-knit communities remind us of the fundamental human need for connection and the joy of being part of a collective.

(opposite) Rural Nicoya

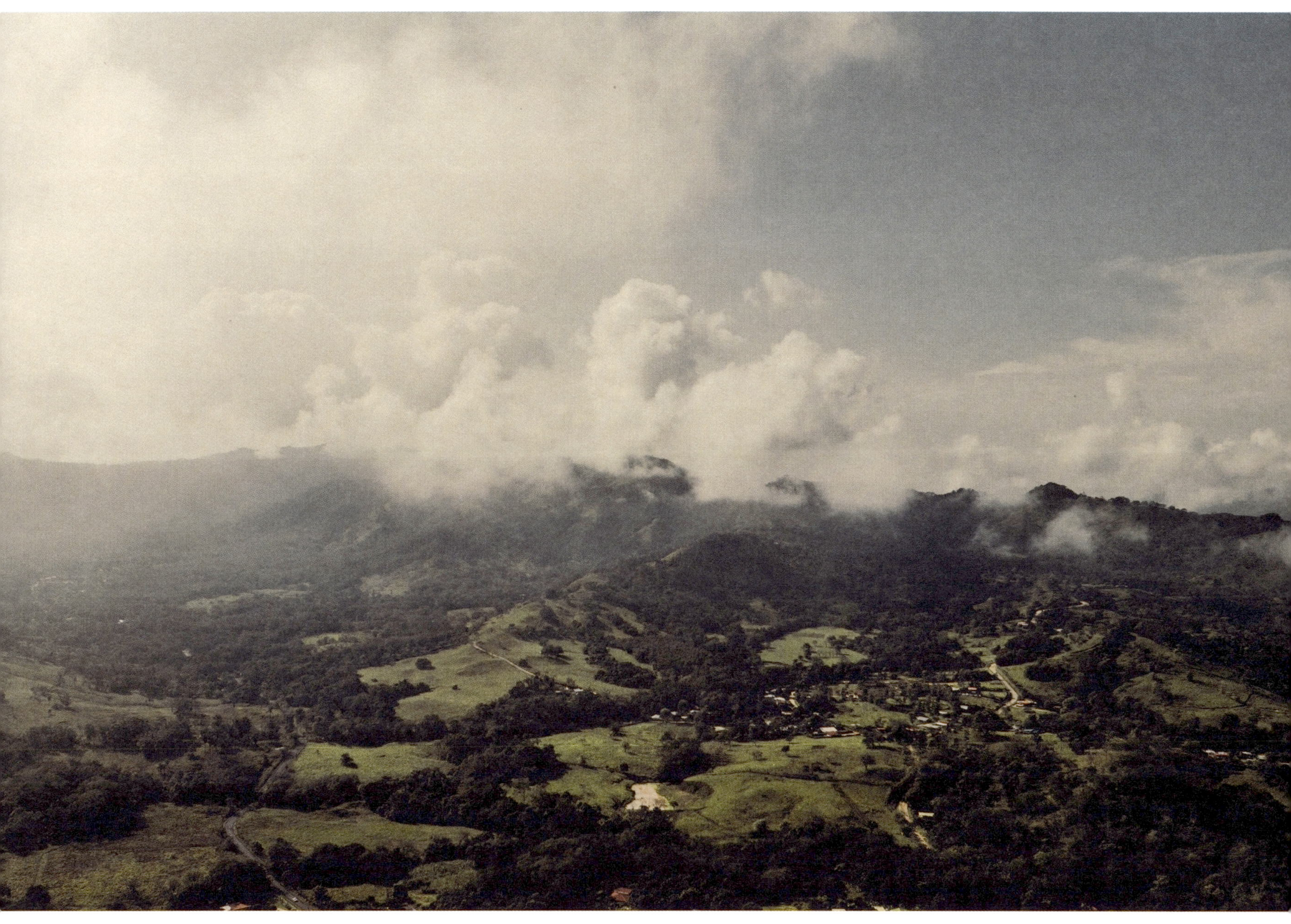

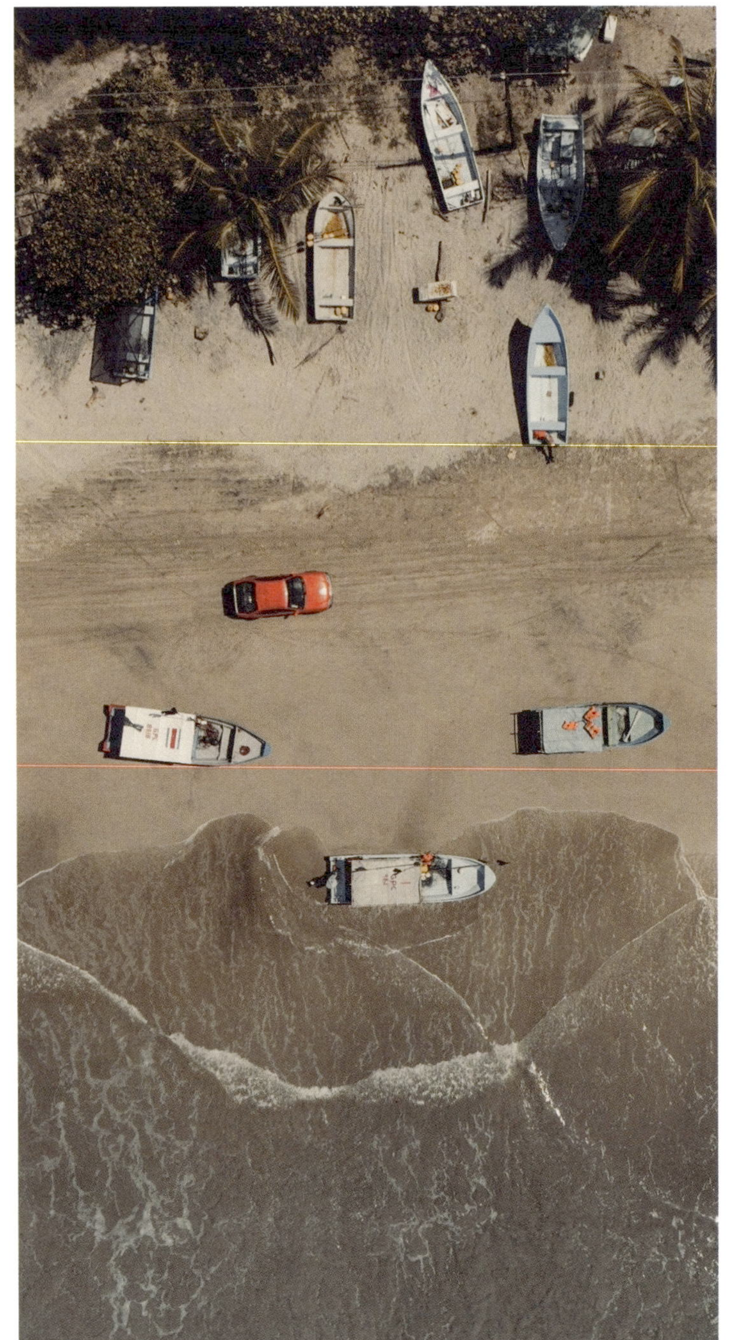

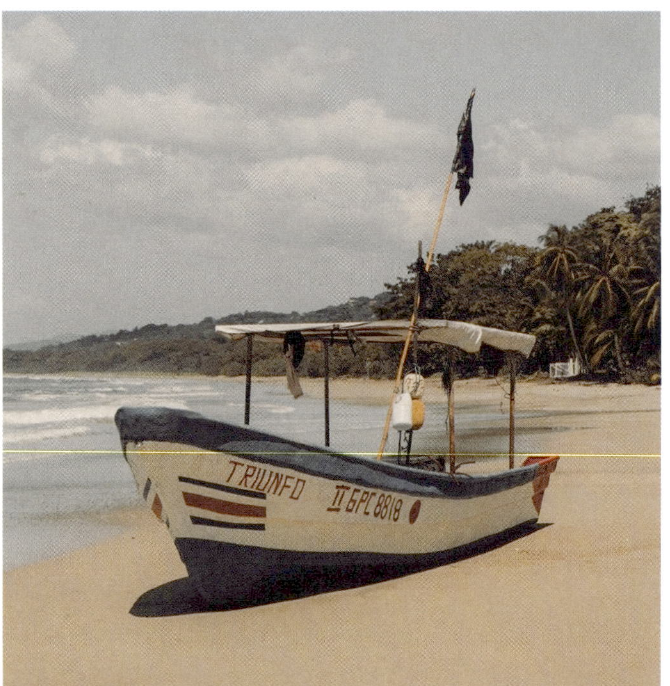

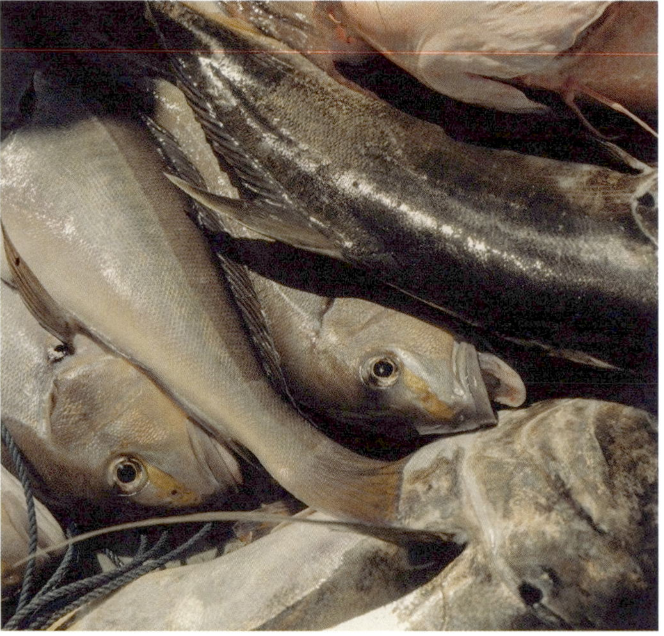

[above left] Beach from above
[above right] Garza fishing boat (top); Local fisherman's catch of the day (bottom)

THE PURA VIDA LIFESTYLE

The elements of the Pura Vida lifestyle reveal that longevity and well-being extend beyond medical advances or material wealth. They highlight the importance of social bonds, purpose, simplicity, respect for elders, and a deep connection to tradition and nature in achieving a holistic and enriching life experience.

COMMUNITY AND FAMILY BONDS: Strong social connections, as seen in the lives of centenarians like Donna Maria, are crucial for emotional and mental health. The deep family ties and community involvement in Nicoya demonstrate the positive impact of belonging and support on longevity.

PURPOSEFUL DAILY LIVING: Engagement in daily activities that are both meaningful and necessary, as exemplified by Ramiro's life, promotes physical and mental agility. The sense of purpose derived from routine tasks and responsibilities contributes significantly to a sense of fulfillment and happiness.

SIMPLICITY AND CONTENTMENT: The modest lifestyle in Nicoya, focused on simple pleasures and basic living, fosters contentment and reduces stress. This simplicity, coupled with a focus on life's essentials like family, food, and community, helps maintain a balanced and joyful life.

RESPECT AND CARE FOR ELDERS: The high regard and care for the elderly, as practised by individuals like Jorge, highlight the importance of integrating seniors into the community. This respect enhances the elders' sense of worth and belonging, contributing to their overall well-being.

CONNECTION TO TRADITION AND NATURE: Traditional practices, such as cooking and agriculture, keep the people of Nicoya connected to their roots and the environment. This connection to nature and heritage plays a vital role in maintaining physical health and a sense of identity.

LIVING THE PURA VIDA LIFESTYLE: TIPS FOR A FULFILLING LIFE

By integrating these practices into your daily routine, you can embrace the essence of the Pura Vida lifestyle, leading to a more balanced, joyful, and fulfilling life.

FOSTER STRONG COMMUNITY CONNECTIONS: Actively engage with your local community and build strong social networks. Attend community events, volunteer, or simply spend time with neighbours. Keep in touch with friends and family so those vital connections stay strong. Strong relationships contribute significantly to emotional well-being and longevity.

FIND JOY IN SIMPLICITY: Embrace a lifestyle that values simplicity over materialism. Focus on the essentials that bring happiness, like spending quality time with family, enjoying nature, or savouring home-cooked meals. This can lead to a more content and stress-free life.

INCORPORATE TRADITION AND NATURE INTO DAILY LIFE: Connect with your cultural roots and the natural world around you. Whether it's gardening, cooking traditional recipes, or practising cultural rituals, these activities can provide a sense of identity and belonging.

LIVE PURPOSEFULLY: Engage in daily activities that give you a sense of purpose, whether it's a hobby, work, or community service. Having a reason to wake up every day can enhance your mental and physical health.

CULTIVATE RESPECT AND CARE FOR THE ELDERLY: Honour and involve the elderly in family and community life. Learn from their experiences and wisdom. This respect not only benefits the elderly but also enriches the younger generations.

PRACTISE MINDFULNESS AND GRATITUDE: Take time each day to practise mindfulness and express gratitude for the simple joys of life. This can be through meditation, keeping a gratitude journal, or simply reflecting on the positive aspects of your day.

OUR VOICES OF LONGEVITY

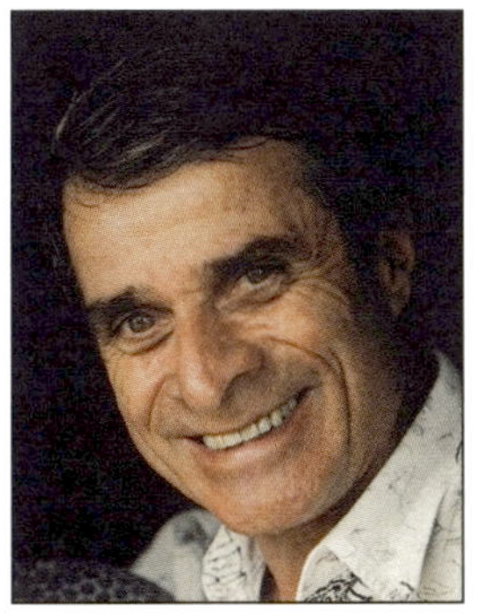

JORGE VINDAS: The heart and soul of the local Blue Zones Association, Jorge is a passionate advocate for the elderly. His journey began with a curiosity about the extraordinary longevity of Nicoya's residents, leading him to dedicate decades to understanding and supporting the region's centenarians, which resulted in the formation of deep, lasting relationships with local elders. Jorge's work extends beyond research; he is a vital part of the community, often seen as a family member by those he assists. His commitment to enhancing the lives of the elderly through his association, which raises funds for those in need, reflects a deep respect and care for the senior population.

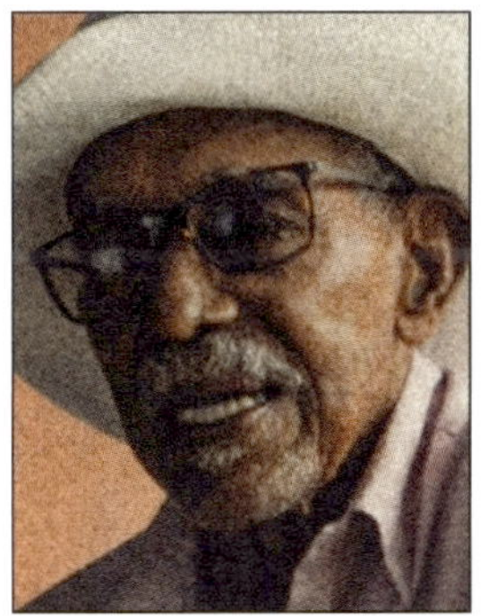

DON RAMIRO: At 102 years old, Ramiro is the epitome of vitality and purposeful living. His daily routine, deeply ingrained in the culture and environment of Nicoya, showcases the extraordinary health and well-being achievable in advanced age. A proud Guanacastean sabanero, Ramiro's lifestyle is a blend of physical activity, social engagement, and a strong sense of identity, which have kept him remarkably fit and mentally sharp. His commitment to purposeful daily tasks, like tending to his cattle and engaging with his community, highlights the importance of staying active and socially connected in promoting quality of life. Ramiro's story challenges conventional views on aging, demonstrating that with the right lifestyle, one's later years can be filled with vigour, purpose, and joy.

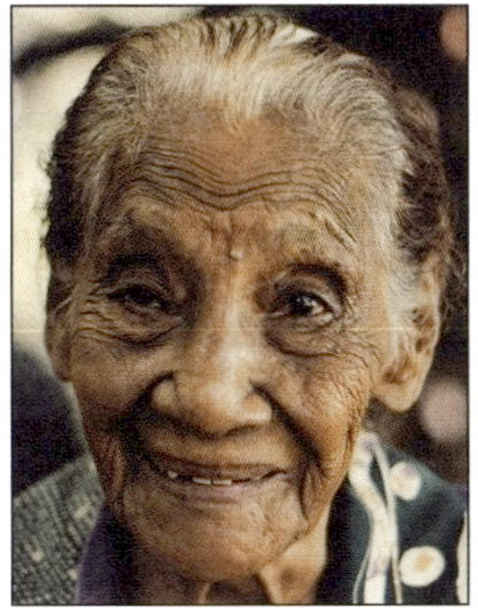

DONNA MARIA: At the heart of Costa Rica's Blue Zone is Donna Maria, a centenarian whose life embodies the essence of the Pura Vida lifestyle. Her simple existence revolves around family, tradition, and the joys of everyday living. At 101, she continues to cook for her family, using traditional methods and recipes passed down through generations. Her life offers a poignant contrast to the often-isolated lives of the elderly in other Western societies. Donna Maria's approach to life, with its emphasis on strong family bonds, communal involvement, and the simple pleasures of daily routines, provides a powerful example of how to live a long, fulfilling life grounded in love, purpose, and connection.

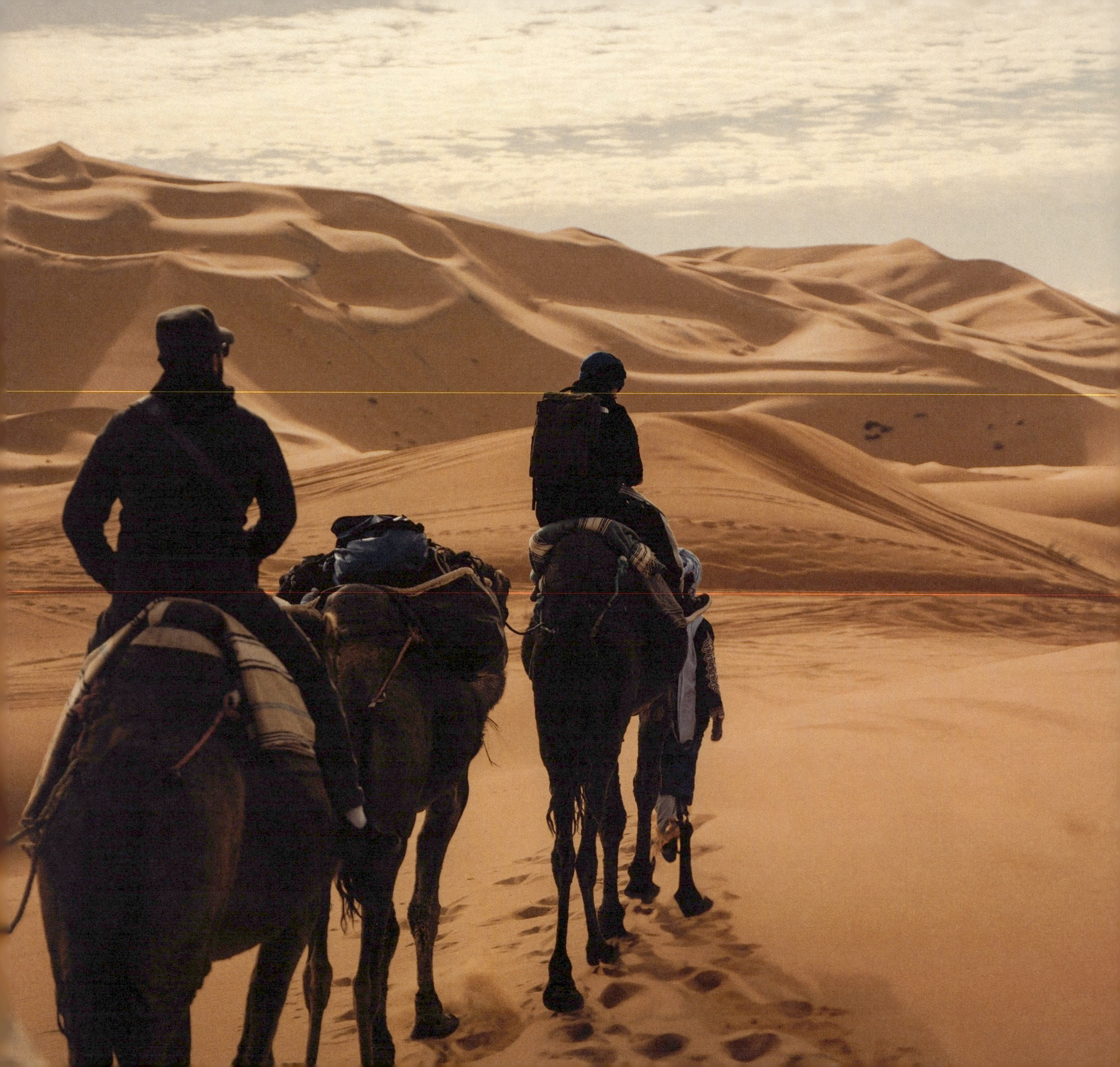

SANDS OF TIME

With its myriad landscapes where resourceful people have lived for millennia, Morocco holds lessons in adaptation. From towering dunes to rugged coastlines, the people of this place embrace traditions that appreciate the moment while heeding the warnings about changing times.

STARING AT STARS

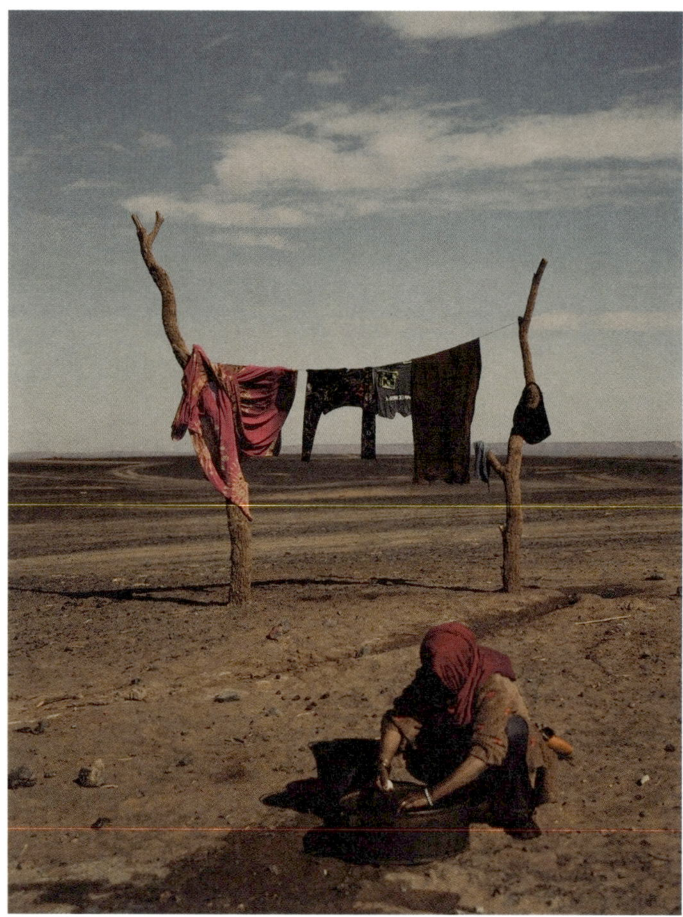

The sun has dipped below the horizon, casting the Sahara into a twilight realm of shifting shadows. Above me, the stars of the Milky Way reveal themselves in the darkening sky like a river of light. In this ocean of sand and stars, I sit on the ridge of a dune, my mind processing the day's journey.

This is my first night in the Sahara. Our three-hour camel trek has brought us to a traditional nomadic tent, a speck of civilization in this silty abyss. The silence is piercing, a complete stillness described to me by my local guide as "the sound of the wind with no wind." The quiet is what strikes me the most. I have never experienced the absence of something so intensely. It is as though this void is an entity that commands your attention without asking for it.

It's a moment of unique reflection, completely contrasting the noisy world I have left behind. I ponder the experiences that led me here—the endless planning, the cultural nuances navigated, the bureaucratic tape of securing film permits. This project, which has taken me across the globe, has placed me here in the darkness of the desert, a place more unfamiliar than any I have ever experienced.

Sitting here, in the vastness of the landscape around me, I am struck by its beauty and nature's incredible talent for mesmerizing. The hush of the Sahara is tangible in its intensity. It is as if the dunes communicate in a language beyond words, telling me to slow down and pay attention to where I am. It's been said that the Sahara speaks to its visitors of ancient memories, resilience, and, like the sands in an hourglass, the passage of time.

Without the sun's encouragement, the sand beneath me is cooling rapidly, and the air has taken on a chill. I can now hear distant laughter from our camp—subtle sounds amplified in the desert's quiet—and although I see the warm flicker of the campfire in the distance, I don't feel compelled to join quite yet.

This moment, isolated in the heart of the Sahara, is a reminder of the journey's essence—not just the physical travel from one place to another, but the opportunity to connect with a place and know it. The Sahara, with its vastness and stillness, is more than just a backdrop; it is a character shaping my perceptions. It whispers introspection and peace, and I quietly observe while it speaks. Satisfied it has made its point, it releases my mind from its grasp and permits me to give in to the comfort of the fire and join the laughter at the camp.

The tranquility of this evening in Africa is a world apart from how this trip started.

[previous page] Into the desert
[above] Nomad life; [opposite] Berber guides in the dunes

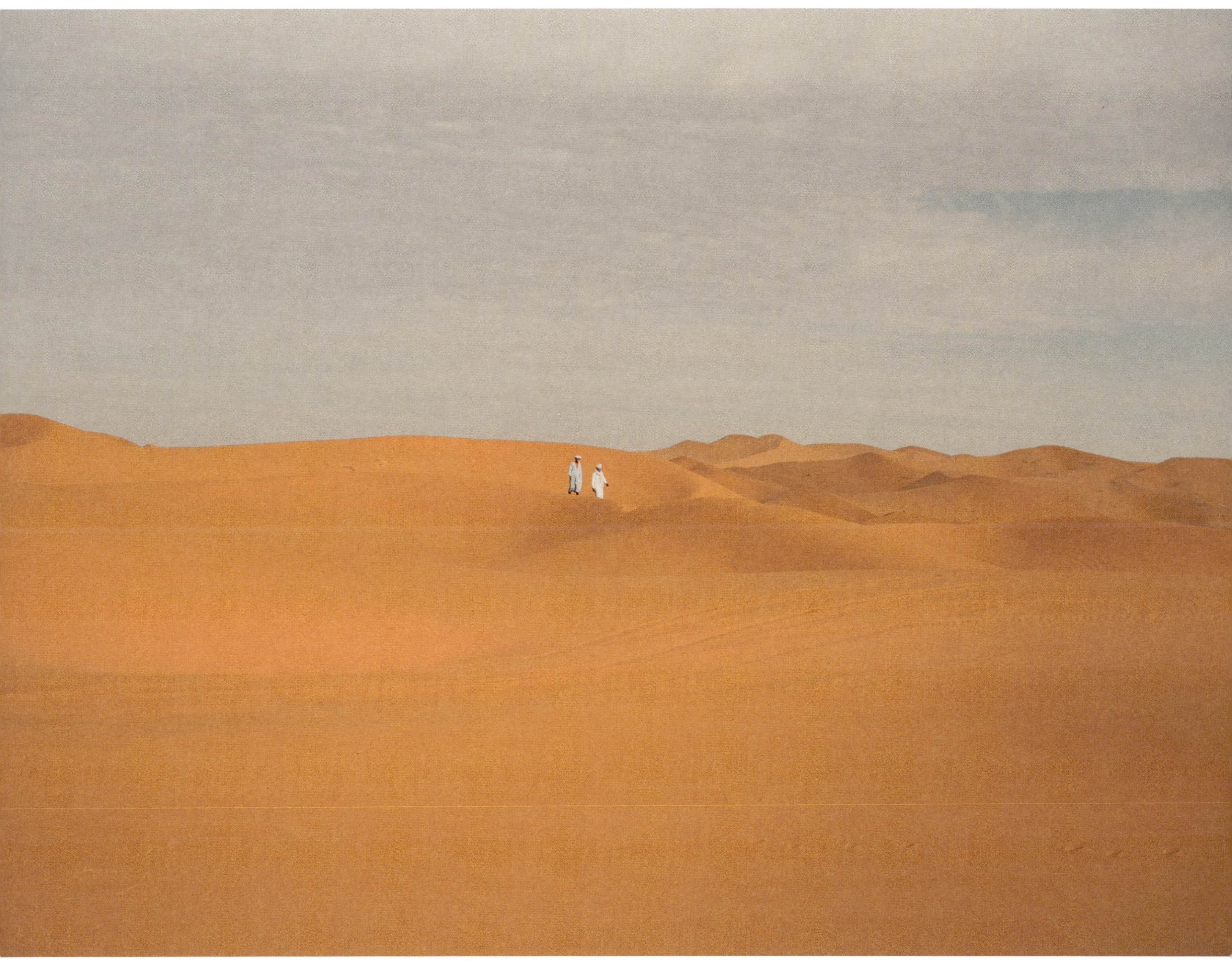

THE JOURNEY

The chaos of a blizzard surrounds the Montreal airport, threatening the entire trip.

I'm anxiously waiting for Braeden, who was stranded in St. John's due to inclement weather there. The only way out was a propeller plane, more adept at handling tricky weather than jets and sought after by experienced Newfoundland travellers. Working like a conductor, I book flights, track planes, and choreograph a route through Halifax to get him to Montreal in time for our flight to Casablanca. The storm outside is relentless. Sitting in the airport, the tension builds with each announcement over the intercom. Finally, Braeden is here, and we board, only to be met with further delays. The plane, queued for de-icing, sits on the tarmac as the minutes turn into hours.

When it's our turn to take off, I catch myself celebrating our departure—too soon. As we speed down the runway, a commotion suddenly breaks out. A passenger, seated just rows behind us, has passed out, and his wife is screaming and attempting to give chest compressions. In a matter of seconds, the cabin transforms from a space of quiet anticipation to one of urgent action. The takeoff is aborted in time, and the man is stabilized, safely offloaded and tended to. And then the waiting begins again. After another round of de-icing, we're ready, and the plane finally takes off, leaving behind a trail of anxiety and relief.

Once we land in Morocco, our challenges are still far from over. Navigating customs proves to be another saga where we are acutely aware of each scrutinizing gaze of the customs officials. Though we have all our film permits in order, the process is a reminder of the complexities involved in international filmmaking.

Then we learn our first guest, crucial to the documentary, cannot meet due to our delay, rendering our first day of shooting a bust.

These initial setbacks, however, do not dampen our spirits. If anything, they strengthen our resolve. I have learned that the road to creating something meaningful is often lined with obstacles. If this is just the start of the trip, then this is shaping up to be an extraordinary adventure.

The following day, we drive from Casablanca to Rabat, where our trip takes a favourable turn. Here, I have the fortune to meet up with my friend Dris, who embodies the essence of Moroccan wellness and shares my enthusiasm for the ocean. Dris, a wellness expert with a broad understanding of Moroccan culture and global wellness trends, had travelled the world before returning to his homeland. His return was motivated by a desire to be closer to his roots and raise his child in Morocco's supportive, community-oriented environment.

Dris' story is compelling. He is a single father of an energetic seven-year-old boy, Noah, whose mother passed at a young age, leaving Dris to take over full-time parenting while balancing work and family. He is not just a wellness expert; he is a student of the field. He and I have shared a similar journey, travelling extensively and learning from diverse cultures. He has now brought his experiences back to Morocco. He is a guide who I hope will help me navigate the deeper layers of Moroccan life and culture.

We arrive at his beach house. Simple and quaint, the house is painted white with blue doors and shutters. The interior is cozy and inviting. An old oil drum has been fashioned into a wood stove, and dry hardwood burns inside. Its radiating heat hits you when you enter the room, holding the salt water dampness

[opposite]
[top] Casablanca sunset; [bottom] The Atlas Mountains

at bay. I'm immediately drawn to the back deck, built into the sand of the Atlantic, where the ocean's giant waves crash against an exposed reef at low tide. Dris shows us around, and we take our respective rooms, eager to get a good night's sleep.

I wake up a few hours later as a chill creeps in from the late-night fog. Instinctively, I move from the bedroom to the couch to sleep in front of the fire, my subconscious drawing on my love of my wood stove at home. I relight the smouldering ashes. The dry wood catches in no time and the crackle of the fire sings me to sleep.

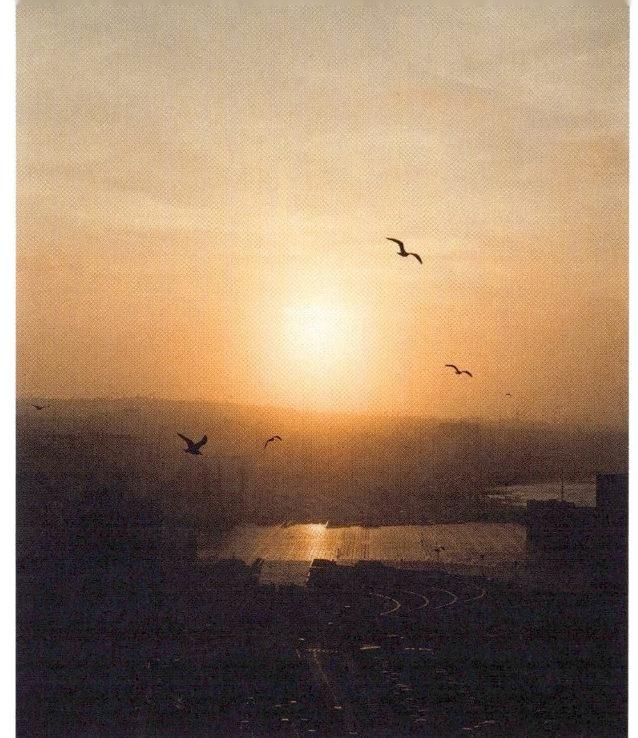

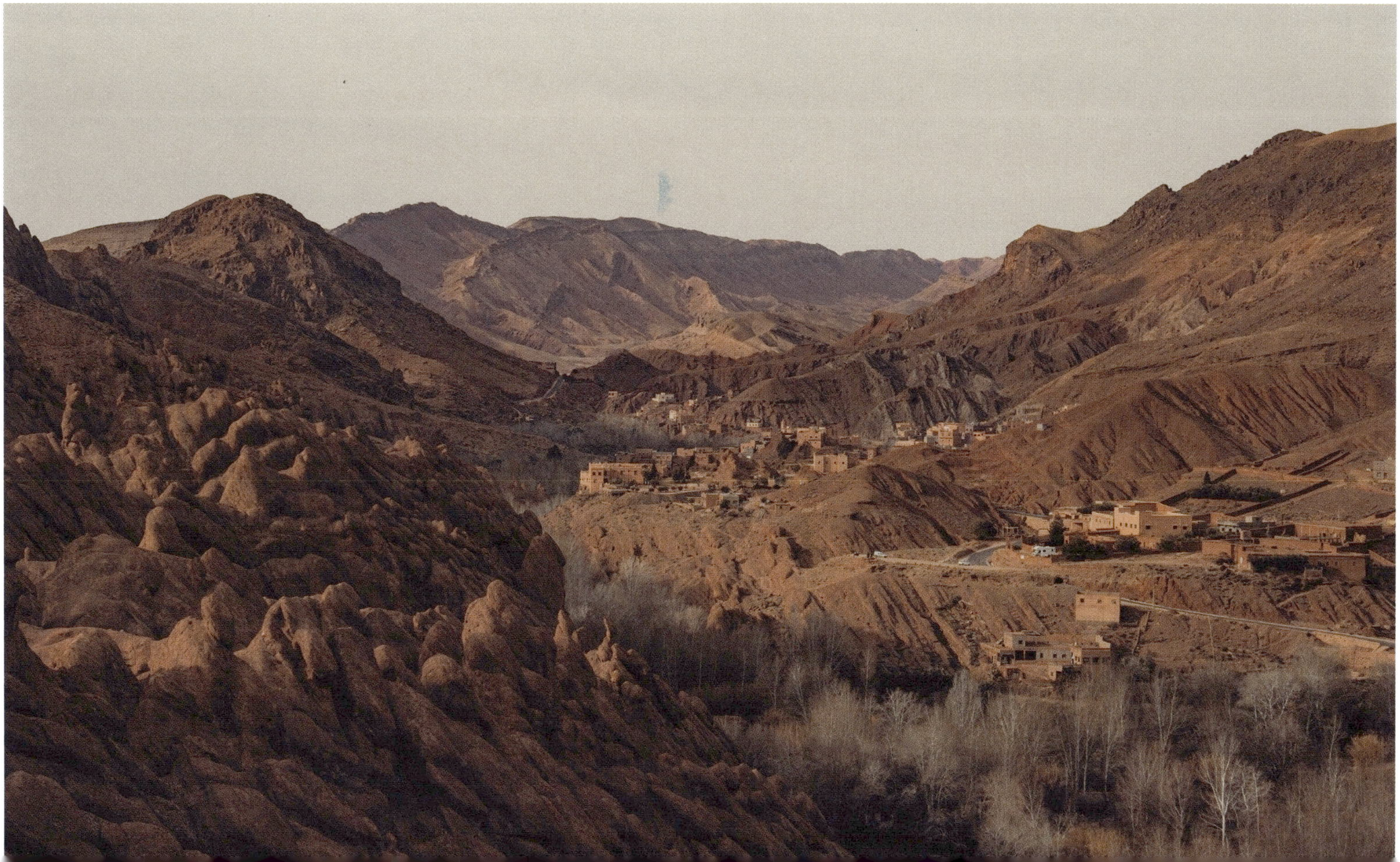

A HOME TO MANY FACES

The following morning, Dris shares his local surf spot with me, so I borrow a wetsuit from his friend who owns the local surf shop. Catching my first waves in Africa is pure joy, even though I can see I am vastly under-skilled as I sit in the lineup watching surfer after surfer take off with perfect form, screaming down the line past a backdrop of beachgoers and Moroccan kasbahs.

Those towering kasbahs are citadels, built of mud and clay and situated harmoniously into the landscape. Designed with strong foundations, many have survived centuries and now draw tourists from around the globe. But I haven't come here for tourist attractions and don't yet know that the kasbah embodies the lessons I will learn about life in Morocco.

I spend time learning from Dris. Our discussions delve into various aspects of Moroccan culture, lifestyle, and the broader concept of wellness. Dris speaks of the importance of community, the value of a slower pace of life, and the deep connection Moroccans have with their land and traditions. These themes resonate with me, highlighting the stark contrast between the frantic pace of our lives back home and the more measured, thoughtful approach to living in Morocco.

Dris speaks from experience. His story of transitioning from a global nomad to a dedicated father while embracing his heritage will stay with me. It reminds me that, regardless of where life takes us, our roots and culture always hold a special place in our hearts.

We wave goodbye to Dris and load up for the trek to Marrakesh. There, we will join three key figures. Khalid, our lead contact, brings a depth of knowledge about Morocco's cultural and environmental landscapes. He has filmed with *National Geographic*, worked with BBC correspondents across Africa, and casually comments that we are the 1128th project he has fixed. Tall and slim in his olive-green work shirt, he has a firm handshake and always carries two cell phones to keep connected. His kindness, thoroughness, and even physical mannerisms trigger thoughts of my father that are impossible to ignore. I wonder what strange sense of humour the universe has, making him the person responsible for our safety.

Ibrahim, a skilled drone pilot, is friendly and fun-loving, and adores his family. We become friends instantly. He is curious about Canada and eager to share photos of his happy three-year-old. He and Braeden quickly begin to talk gear and check out the three drones he brought.

I stroll over to introduce myself to Samad, our driver, as he smokes a Camel cigarette beside our black Land Cruiser. Never without his dark aviator sunglasses, he prides himself on his driving playlist, which is filled with funky North African music—artists that are new to me. His hands are adorned with silver Berber rings, and his collar is always popped. He reminds me of a Moroccan Elvis Presley in his prime.

We leave the Las Vegas–esque city of Marrakesh to head toward the mountains. Every five minutes, the landscape changes, from plateaus to tree-covered mountains to rocky cliffs to arid valleys.

Even the mountains transform from high peaks to sharp ledges and weather-rounded mounds. As we traverse the winding roads of the Atlas Mountains, the initial reason for my visit—to witness the impact of climate change—becomes increasingly evident. The once mighty rivers carved through

[opposite] Happy campers—Khalid and Ibrahim

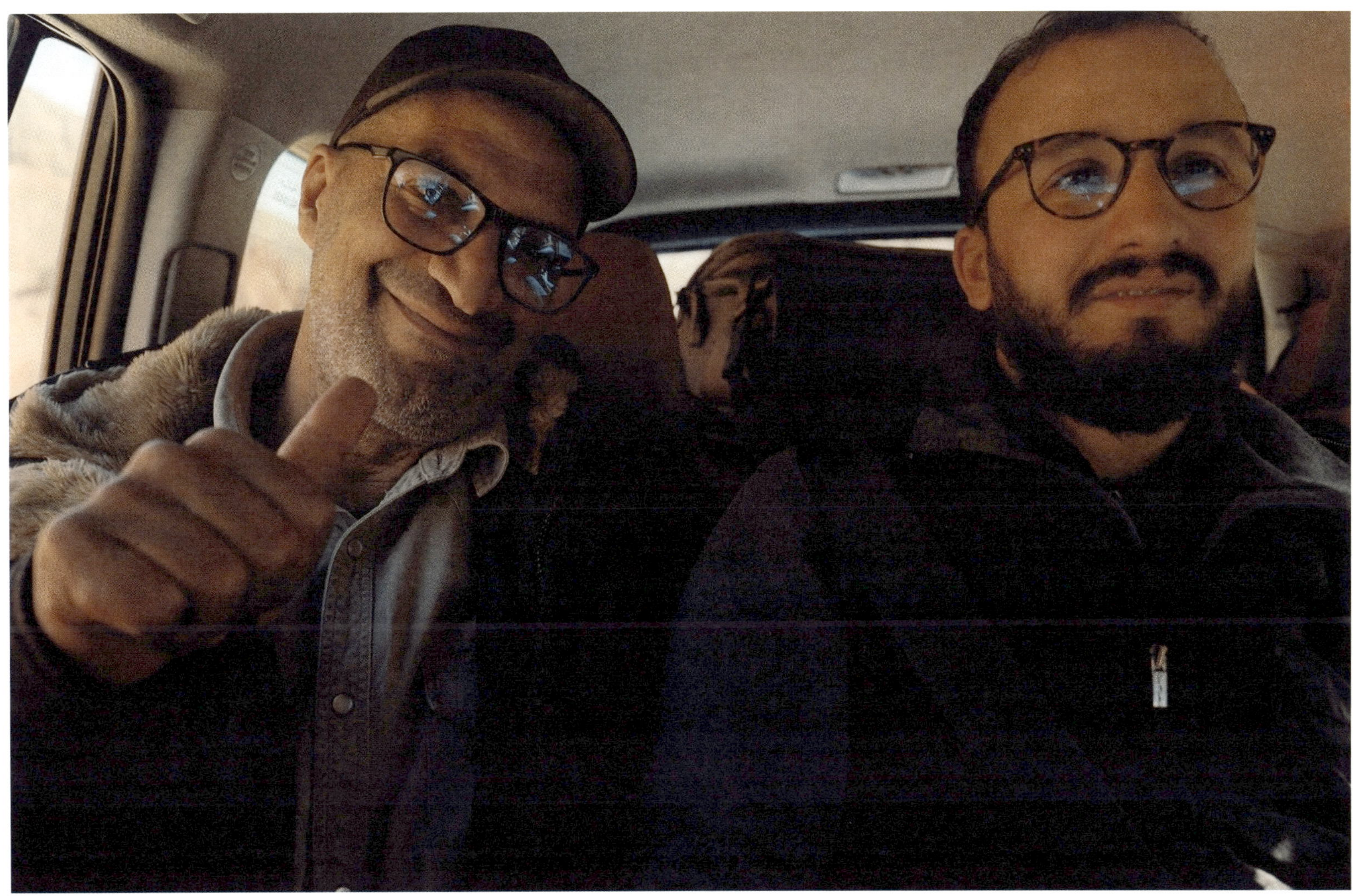

these mountains have been reduced to mere trickles. The sight of these dry riverbeds was a poignant reminder of the fragility of our environment. It brought home the reality of the environmental crises we often hear about but rarely witness firsthand.

The Moroccan team shares their personal experiences and insights about these changes, offering a local perspective on environmental issues. They tell me that the snow from the high Atlas Mountains is disappearing, and the downstream effects are being felt. This is the rainy season, but I would never know; there isn't a cloud in the sky, and we haven't seen a drop of rain since we arrived. We drive all day, and although the distance travelled isn't far, the windy roads inch us toward the south of the country. We stay in the mountains this evening. The chill of the high mountain air creeps into our bones as we unload the truck. It is just above zero degrees Celsius, and the air is crisp, but the room is warm and heat flows from the furnace.

INTO THE DESERT

We wake up before the sun and grab a quick breakfast before loading the truck and heading out of the mountains as the sun peeks over the rocky horizon. Switchback after switchback, we drive the famous Dadès Gorge, which could rival the Grand Canyon. Emerging from the base of the high peaks, the scenery flattens out almost immediately. The desert has begun—a rocky, barren surface that triggers thoughts of Mars. There is no life here, a wasteland of dirt, and as we drive the seemingly endless road, a golden vision appears on the horizon. The landscape transforms before my eyes as we approach the distant banks. The infinite expanse of golden dunes, shaped and reshaped by the winds, presents the Sahara's stark beauty.

We arrive at our meeting point, where three Berber men with six camels are waiting. It's getting late in the day, and we have a three-hour trek, atop camels, as darkness falls over the desert.

Camels aren't small—they are enormous. Thankfully, they kneel down for us to load our gear onto before we climb aboard. I name mine JP—short for Jean Pierre, an homage to the French heritage of Morocco and in honour of an old Acadian friend. Hammou, our guide, signals the camel to stand up and tells me to hold on tight. I follow the advice and grip the metal saddle as hard as possible. As the beast's hind legs extend, I am thrown forward like an amusement ride. It's an unexpected rush. JP then moves to his front knees and then hooves and I am up—up almost three metres in the air!

Then we are off. It's ironically anticlimactic and wildly slow. My concerns over ensuring we capture enough footage of the camels proves to be a ridiculous underestimation of opportunity as we have several hours each day on these animals. The slow and steady pace of the camels contrasts sharply with the hectic speed of our previous travels, and with this newfound time, I begin to focus on the moment. Riding atop these strange creatures, we lumber through the rolling dunes, each step taking us deeper into the heart of the desert. The journey, though physically uncomfortable at times, is a meditative experience. Each dune is unique, and it holds your mind until thoroughly studied.

The sun is now well below the horizon and all that remains is the golden line of the day that was. We round a dune and I realize we have arrived at our campsite. The camels drop to their knees, and I navigate the descent with a firm grip on the saddle. There is a solitary black desert tent in a valley of dunes, but within minutes, the site springs to life as rugs are pulled out and a fire is started. As soon as the coals glow red, it is time for us to be introduced to an integral part of Moroccan culture: the tea-making ritual. We drank tea with several people along the road, but it was already prepared. Now I see that brewing tea is not a simple act; it involves ceremony that takes time and cannot be rushed.

The tea preparation is meticulous, a custom that involves boiling the water and adding green tea leaves, fresh mint, and a generous amount of sugar to the teapot.

The tea pouring is an art performed with grace and precision, transforming the process into a captivating performance. A series of small glasses are set out to receive, and the pour begins at the rim of the glass, but as the stream of tea appears from the spout, the pot is lifted about a metre into the air. The trick is to get as high as possible, as quickly as possible, before the glass is filled

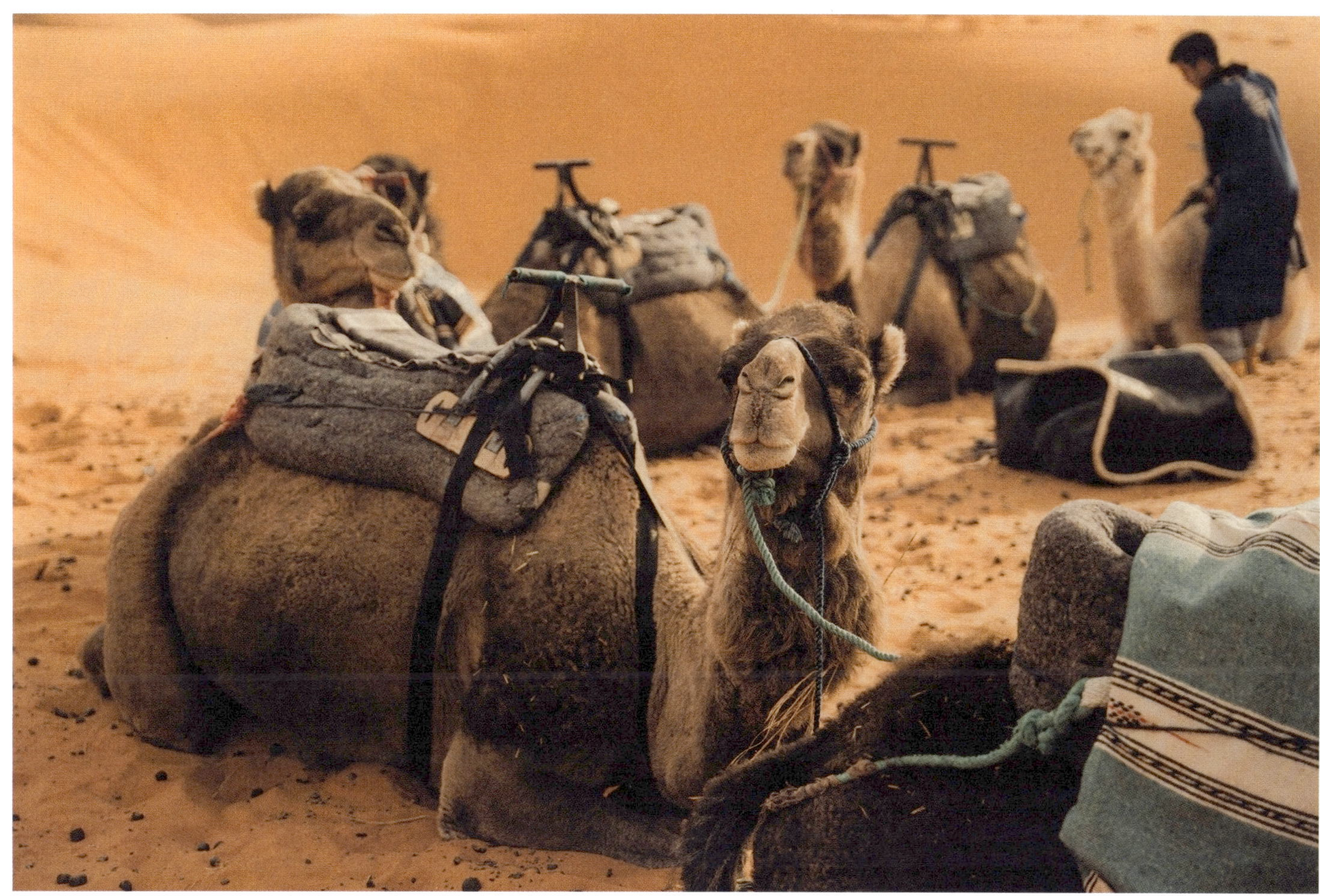

while not spilling any tea. Once several tea glasses have been poured, the pot is placed down, and the top is opened. The tea is poured back into the pot, and then the process is repeated up to four or five times.

There is a reason for repetition outside of its theatrical marvel.

The foam on the top of Moroccan tea, which appears after the dramatic pour, is like the "crema" of coffee. I learn that this foam is considered a sign of a well-made tea, indicating that it has been properly brewed and aerated. As I try my hand at pouring the tea, I am told that pouring from a height not only cools the tea slightly, making it more immediately drinkable, but also aerates it, enhancing its flavour and creating the desirable foam on top. But pouring from a height is a practiced skill that illustrates the pourer's proficiency. Inspecting the glass I poured, the foam is noticeably absent and tea has been spilled. Graciously, my hosts say well done but in the same motion, quickly take the teapot from me before I try my hand again.

"Why tea instead of coffee?" The answer, I'm told, is simple. Coffee is made quickly and gives us instant energy. Tea, on the other hand, takes time to prepare and is made for sipping. You also don't just have one tea when you arrive somewhere; you are expected to have two, maybe three glasses. Tea is

[above] Camels taking a break

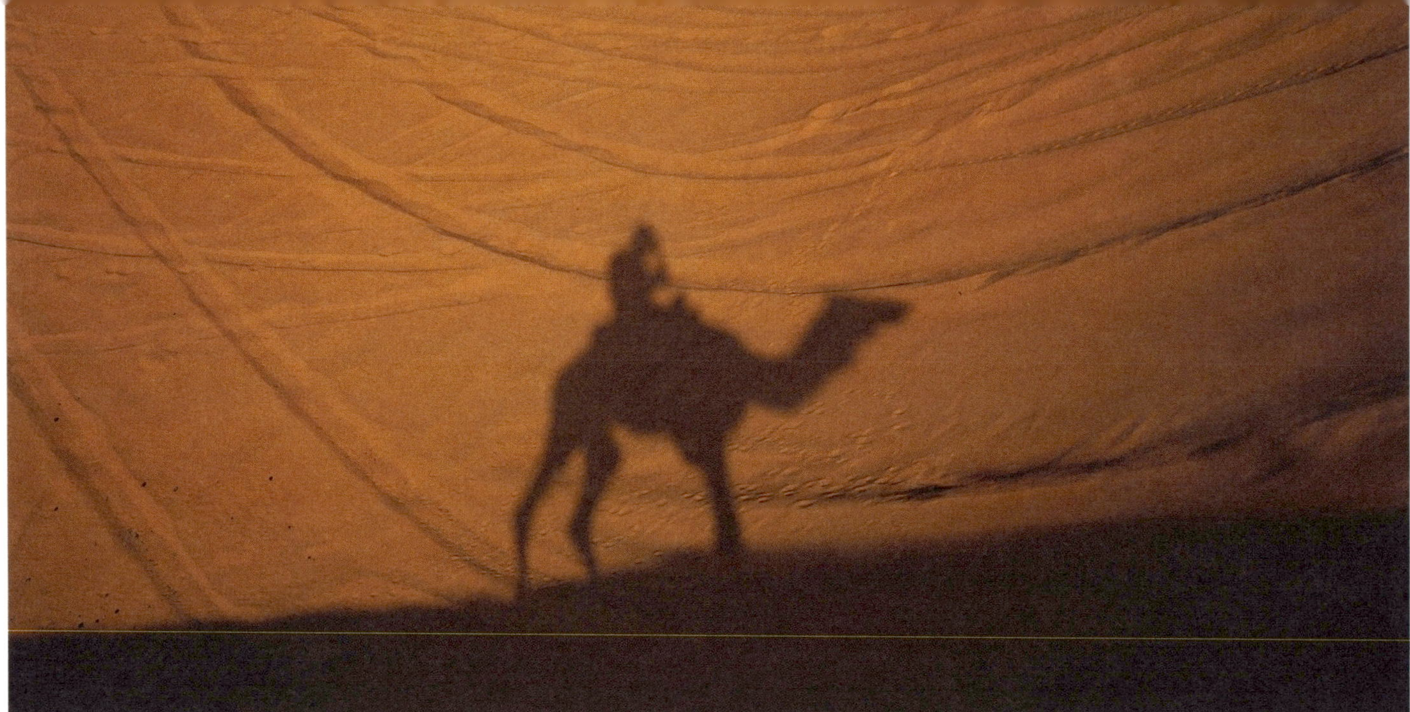

synonymous with dialogue, connection, and an expectation of attentiveness. This tradition is about more than just making tea; it is about creating a space for conversation and sharing stories and experiences. In Morocco, tea symbolizes hospitality and friendship; it's how business is done and provides a way to respect someone by enjoying their tea and offering your time.

After tea, it's time for a communal meal that provides further insight into Moroccan life. I am introduced to tagine, a culinary staple of Moroccan cuisine. A tagine pot features a distinctive shape that emphasizes cooking functionality. It consists of two parts: a broad, shallow, circular base designed for evenly spreading ingredients, which later becomes the dish the meal is served on, and a unique cone- or dome-shaped lid that sits atop the base. This lid is designed to condense steam and return it to the dish and has a small hole in the top. I am told that this ensures food remains moist and flavourful. The dish we are using is made of clay, and since food is slow-cooked, it tenderizes meats the same way a braise might.

Preparing the meal is a communal activity, with each ingredient carefully added, layer by layer, into the pot. First, it's onions and garlic, followed by seasoned chicken. Then, we create a cone-shape around the chicken that will follow the shape of the tagine lid, placing sliced potatoes, carrots, eggplant, and cucumber and topping the mountain of food with tomatoes. Handfuls of Moroccan spice is added. The lid is placed on top, and the tagine is cooked over an open fire of coals. I take this opportunity to head up to the dune to stare at the stars, and when I return, we gather around the roaring fire and share stories of our homes. The warmth of the fire and the aroma of the cooking food are comforting, and for a moment, I forget we are in the middle of the desert. We are all sprawled out on our respective blankets and stare into the fire. No one is forcing conversation, and the evening flows as our dinner cooks. In this place, it feels as if time is elastic and endless.

After about an hour and a half, the meal is ready to eat, and we sit around a small round table, tearing off bread and using it to take up big chunks of chicken, veggies, and the gravy made at the bottom of the dish. It is strangely similar to the Newfoundland "cooked dinner": a boiled dish made each Sunday with meat and veggies, salt and spices.

The vastness of the desert and the endless canopy of stars invite me to let go of my worries. As we all share stories and food, and drink tea, the superficial differences that often divide people of distinctive cultures disappear, revealing our fundamental human connections.

When I tuck in for the night under the camel-hair tent, I pull up two heavy wool blankets to stay warm. The sand under me moulds to my body, and I drift off, full and content.

[above] Shadows on the sand

TAKING TIME

The dawn in the Sahara is a spectacle that defies description. As the first rays of the sun peek over the horizon, the desert is bathed in a soft, warm light. With their sharp contours and shadows, the dunes transform into an opus of oranges, pinks, and yellows.

We emerge from our tents into crisp and cool air, a refreshing change from the previous day's heat and the night's freeze. Wrapped in our jackets, we watch in awe as the sun ascends, its warmth gradually infusing the desert with its light. The sunrise over the dunes is mesmerizing and something I will never erase from my memories. I imagine this must be how people see a fresh snowfall for the first time, and then smile when I realize how far I am from the familiar.

Today, we ride several hours to visit a nearby nomad camp. This visit is integral to my journey, offering a glimpse into a vastly different lifestyle. The nomadic people of the Sahara have a unique way of life, intricately tied to the rhythms and moods of the desert.

As we approach the camp, the sight of the nomads' tents, crafted from woven fabrics and strategically placed to withstand the desert elements, is a shocking reminder of how differently people live. Their tents, tattered and patched with clothing, are the simplest of dwellings. Even after all my travels, I am shocked by the minimalistic means by which they live. The nomads welcome us with open arms, their hospitality generous and sincere despite their modest means.

For millennia, their life has been a dance of movement and adaptation, following the rains and the seasons, always in sync with the natural world. It's a life of simplicity yet rich in knowledge and wisdom passed down through generations. Home is a series of small tents—one for socializing, another for sleep, one as a kitchen and another as a storage space. A small herd of goats just to the side of the camp grazes in what looks like rocks, not grass. I meet the lady of the house as she prepares what is known to locals as madfouna, or colloquially as Berber pizza, a combination of bread and veggies. I would describe it as more of a veggie calzone than a pizza, but I see the resemblance. The small kitchen is stifling in the desert heat as the fire of the small mud stove roars with the dry tinder she supplies. In the socializing tent, Hammou prepares tea. Before long, the food is ready and served with a heaping bowl of local couscous and salted beef. The meal is simple but hearty, and although I instinctively worry about my Western stomach handling the foods, the only side effect is a full and contented belly.

During the meal, we chat with the nomads and learn they no longer migrate with the rains. The rains have stopped, and the government now brings them water. Their purpose and way of life is gone like the water, and there are fewer of them all the time. With no education or skills to work outside of the desert, many send their children away to school to be educated. These are some of the last nomads of the Sahara, and I am lucky to spend the day learning about their way of life before it is gone.

On our last night in the desert, we stay at a permanent base of tents. In the evening, I notice Khalid sitting by himself in the large tent in the compound's centre. I head over to see him and end up in a conversation that encapsulates my entire journey in Morocco.

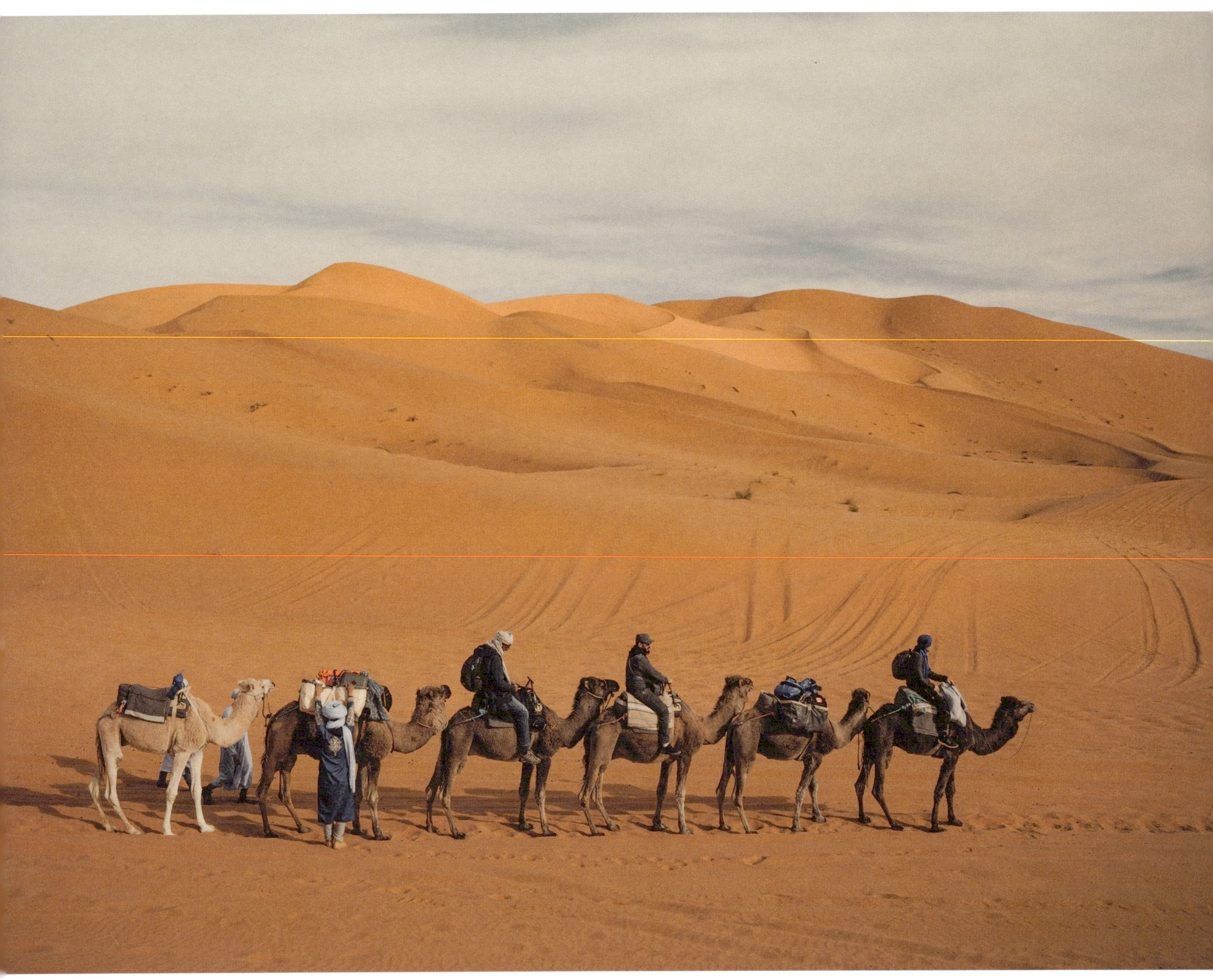

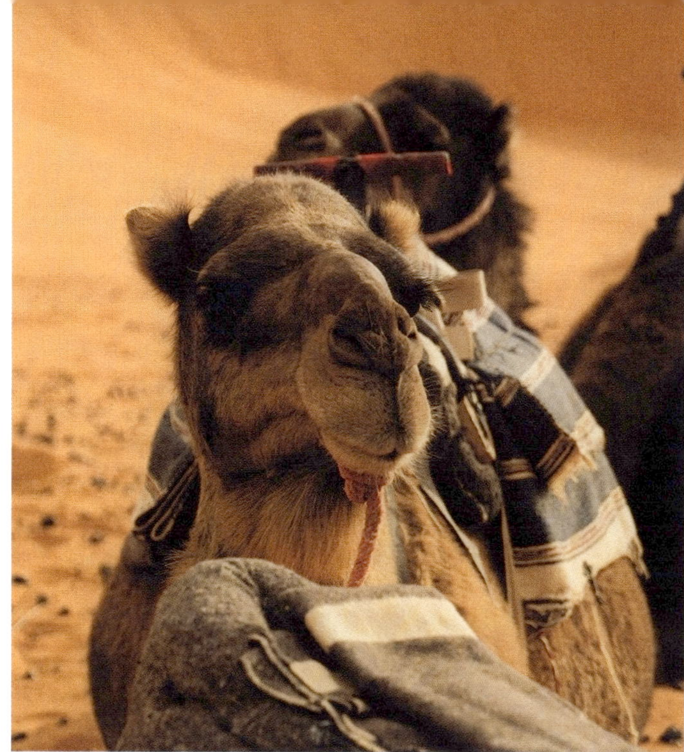

As I sit across from Khalid in the dimly lit glow of our tent, he pours me a cup of tea and we begin to talk. For the next two hours, our conversation unfolds in a way that feels less like a simple discussion and more like a lesson from a wise sage. Khalid has experienced the depths of human existence in a world vastly different from my own back home. His stories, rich with wisdom and ease, offer glimpses into a life lived fully and deeply. He speaks of the world in its myriad forms, each tale imbued with intentional wisdom.

Eventually the topic shifts to the essence of storytelling. Khalid articulates something I've always sensed but have never fully been able to express—the immense power of genuine narratives born from real, unfiltered experiences. His words resonate deeply, affirming my belief in sharing stories with authenticity.

"The key," Khalid says, his eyes reflecting the lantern's flicker, "is to capture stories with genuine curiosity, untainted by what we expect to find." His hands gesture with a large arc as he speaks, emphasizing the importance of telling the whole story as it happens, free from preconceived notions and biases.

This idea strikes a chord in me, and a sense of reassurance washes over me. In my journey of learning, I've always sought to unravel stories in their truest sense, uncoloured by my expectations. It has been in those diversions that the joy of my travels has revealed itself.

Our conversation naturally shifts to the broader implications of our work. Health, as he describes it, is a tapestry woven from threads of culture, environment, and personal perspectives. I agree, sharing that I feel it is far removed from the sterile confines of textbooks and lecture halls that dominate health education. His perspective mirrors the ethos of my travels, where health was explored as a lived experience, a journey through diverse human and natural landscapes.

As the night deepens, our dialogue meanders through various topics, but a singular theme emerges and stays with me—the importance of taking time—time to learn and time to listen. In the stillness of the Sahara, away from the constant bombardment of digital distractions and the relentless pace of modern life, the value of time becomes overwhelmingly apparent. The deepest learning and understanding occurs in these unhurried conversations and in the moments shared with people like Khalid, Dris, the nomads, and the many others we met.

Khalid's voice lingered: "The greatest lessons often come from the simplest moments." This truth had been evident throughout our journey in Morocco. "If you are in a rush, then you are already dead."

In the desert's silence, with the vast sky above and the ancient sands below, I realize this journey was an exploration of life, not just the environment. Morocco taught me to embrace each experience with curiosity, seek knowledge with mind and heart, and cherish the irreplaceable richness of human connections.

Khalid pours me another cup of tea, and we hear a drumbeat starting around the fire. "We better not miss the fun," he says as he stands up. Agreeing, I extend my hand to shake his. "Thank you," I say. A simple acknowledgement that his message hit, and that the moment was not wasted.

"You're welcome." He smiles as we grab our fresh cups of tea and make our way to the rhythm of the drums.

[opposite] The Caravan
[above] Desert transportation

KASBAHS OF HEALTH

In the heart of Morocco, the kasbah stands as a testament to longevity, community, and tradition. IIn the heart of Morocco, the kasbah stands as a testament to longevity, community, and tradition. These fortified structures, with their strong foundations and corner towers, demonstrate balance, function, and simplicity. The kasbah is a metaphor for creating our own fortress of health and an approach to living that can stand the test of time.

THE FOUNDATION—HARMONY WITH NATURE AND TRADITION: Just as a kasbah is built to blend with and withstand the desert around it, our lives should be integrated with our environment and those we live with. Whether it's the traditions surrounding Moroccan tea or the respect for the dunes of the Sahara, we can find harmony almost anywhere. Nature heals our physical and spiritual well-being, grounding us in its presence. Prioritize time to immerse yourself in your environment, wherever you live. Spending time in nature provides space and connection to your surroundings and fosters an appreciation for your home.

FIRST TOWER—COMMUNITY AND SOCIAL BONDS: The first tower stands for community strength and connection, much like the social spaces within a kasbah where guests are greeted. Moroccan culture emphasizes sharing food, moments, and hospitality and forging strong social bonds. These relationships act as keystones in our lives that this tower can be built on. Incorporate this into your life by being generous with your time and space. Invite friends for a meal, offer help without expecting anything in return, and create an inviting atmosphere in your home to foster deeper connections.

SECOND TOWER—PURPOSEFUL ENGAGEMENT: The second tower represents purposefully engaging with your surroundings. The kasbah is central to the success of a community and provides direction for its people. Be purposeful in engaging and learning from local customs. Make an effort to strengthen your bonds with family, friends, and neighbours. Attend community events, support local businesses, and engage in activities that bring people together to build a sense of belonging and support. Most importantly, live with intention and purpose while seeking meaningful growth and community health.

THIRD TOWER—SIMPLICITY AND PRESENCE: The third tower embodies simplicity and the art of being present. The kasbah is built with available materials; it is humble in design yet functional. Appreciate life's simple pleasures, be content with what you have, and seek balance instead of tipping the scales of accomplishment, wealth, or "having more." True wealth lies in a life well lived. Whether it's a few minutes of meditation, a walk in nature, or simply sitting in stillness, these moments can help you connect more deeply with yourself and others.

FOURTH TOWER—VALUING TIME: The fourth tower represents valuing time and the art of being present, reflecting the kasbah's enduring nature. This principle, woven into the fabric of Moroccan life, reminds us of the importance of how we spend our time and the quality of our attention. Prioritizing meaningful interactions, savouring moments, and being fully present fortify our well-being and deepen our connections with others. Focus on what truly matters: relationships, experiences, and personal growth. Declutter your physical and digital spaces, prioritize activities that bring you joy and fulfillment, and practise feeling gratitude for the simple pleasures in life

OUR MOROCCAN MESSENGERS

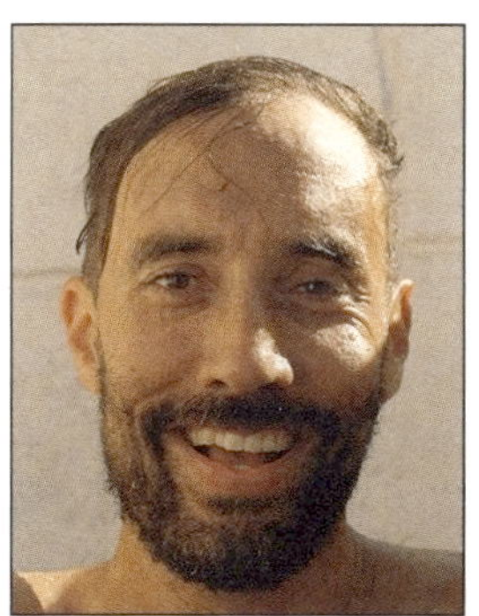

DRIS: Our Moroccan wellness guide, Dris, encapsulates a blend of global perspectives and cultural traditions. His return home to raise his son, Noah, in a community-oriented environment demonstrates the impact of the people we connect with as we grow. He has lived a life emphasizing the importance of community support, the richness of cultural identity, and the benefits of integrating global wellness practices into our daily lives.

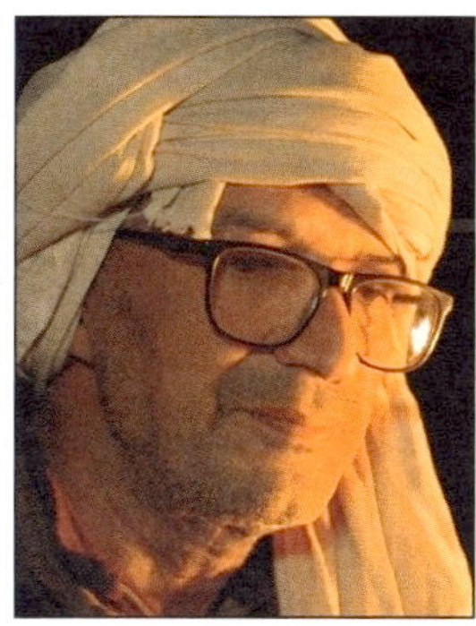

KHALID: Our other Moroccan guide represents the importance of storytelling and cultural preservation. His career has included sharing Morocco's stories with the world and being a custodian of Morocco's heritage through media. He reminds us to prioritize authenticity and truth in our missions and that our personal and collective histories are the threads that weave together the fabric of society and our relationships with one another.

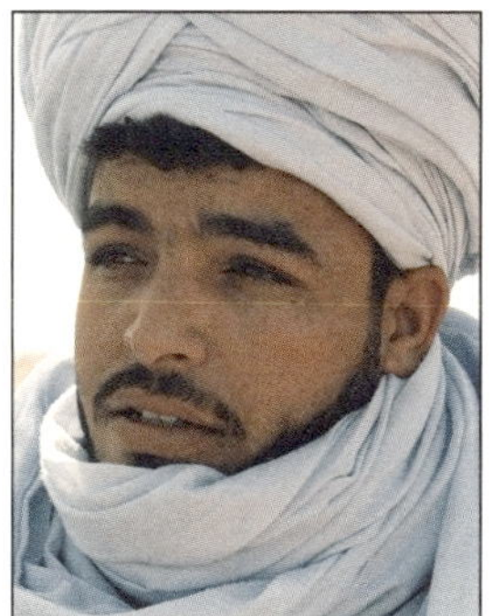

THE NOMADS: The lives and traditions of the nomadic families of the Sahara have been shaped by their environment but are now altered by the changing climate. Once these peoples thrived through their interdependence with the desert, but that way of life is no longer sustainable. They may have been among the first communities to be impacted, but they will not be the last. Their story urges us to embrace sustainability and adaptability because time is running out.

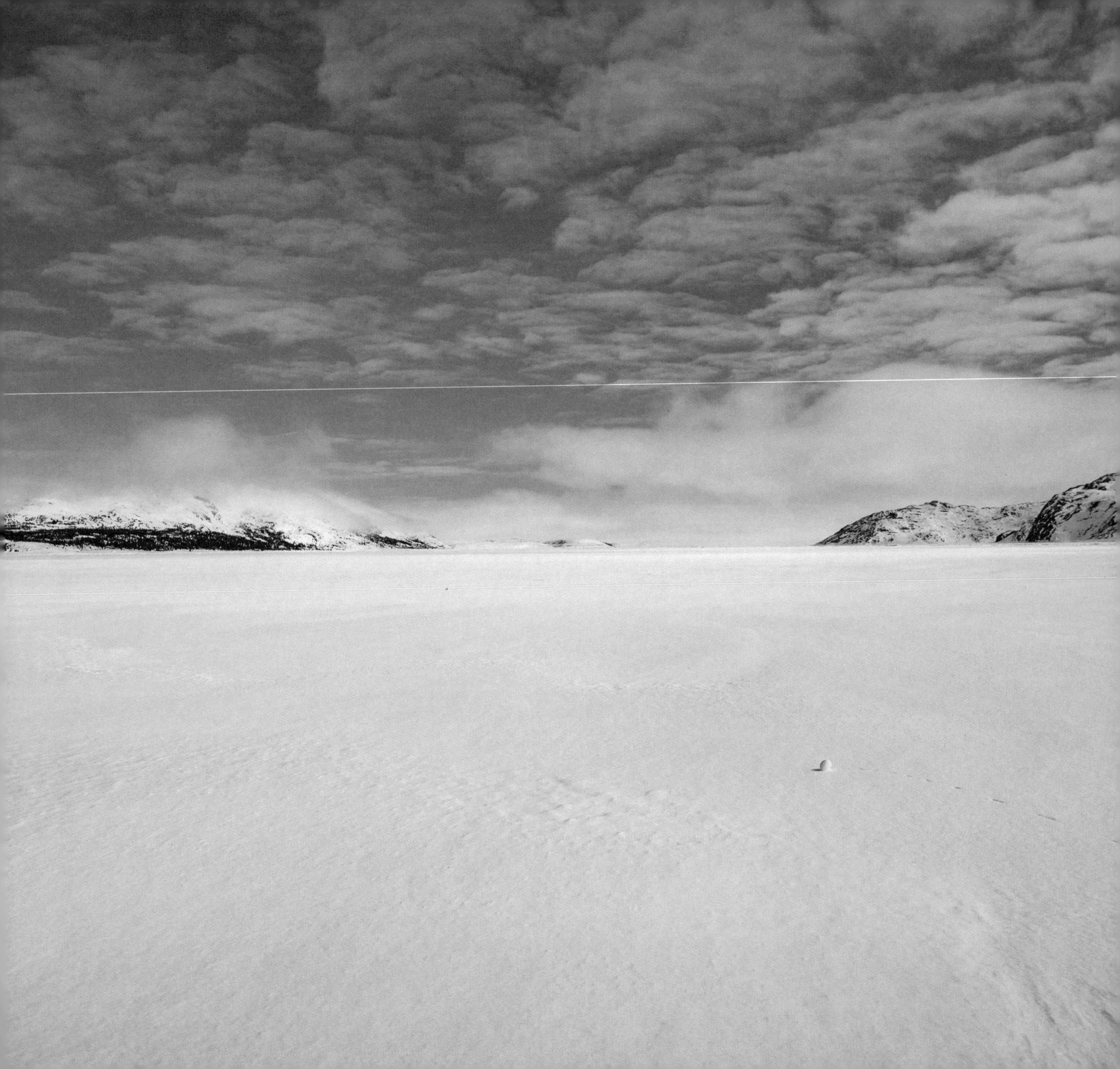

ON THIN ICE

In the stark beauty of Northern Labrador, the melting ice reveals a dire warning. As the climate changes, it threatens the health and way of life for some of the most vulnerable members of our community. It took this visit to the north of my own province to teach me how the health of our planet is synonymous with the health of the people who live on it.

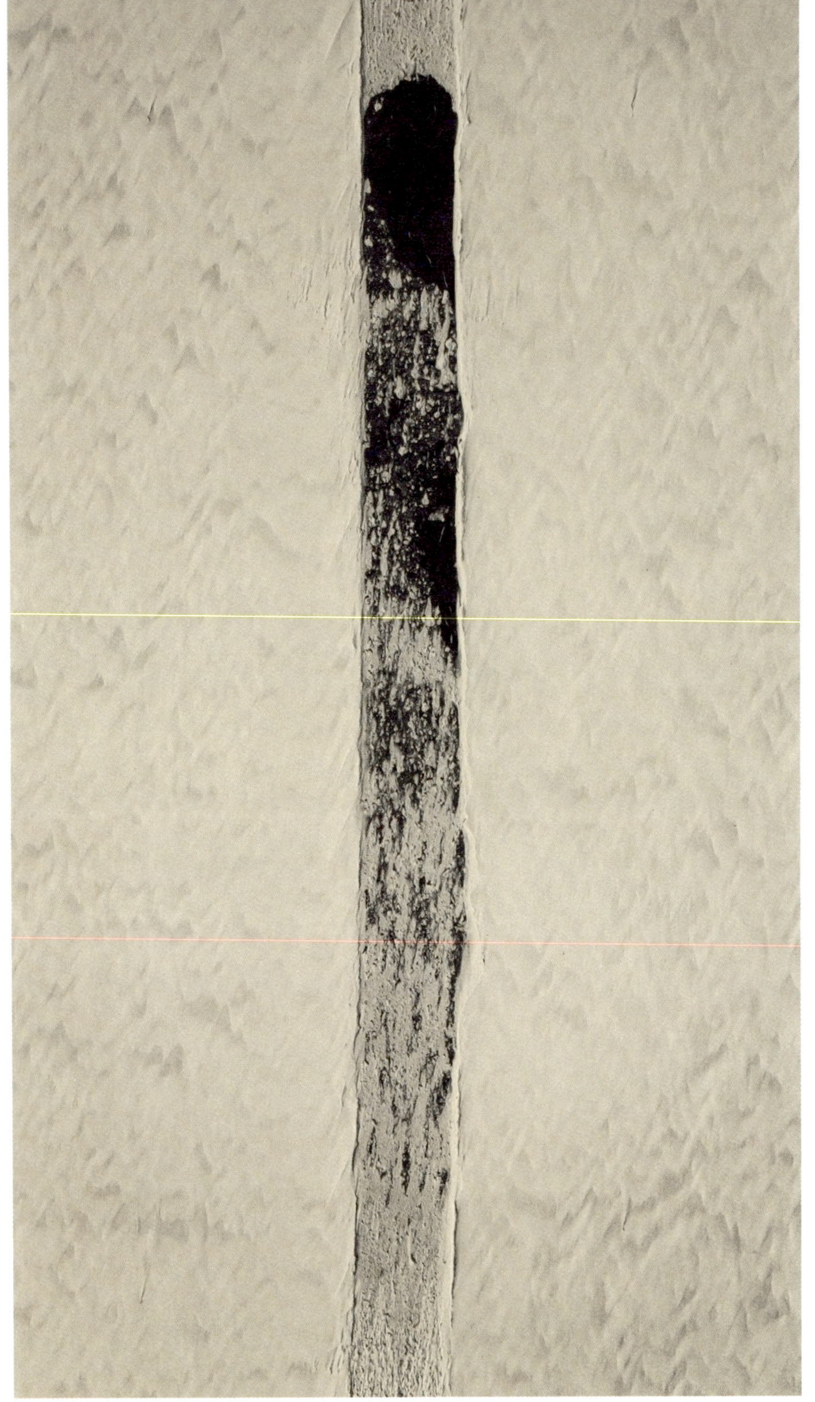

As our small twin-engine prop plane descends through the low cloud cover, the town of Nain appears beneath us like a mystical realm. Shrouded in the rugged coast of Northern Labrador, it is encased in a silent white canvas.

ARCTIC ARRIVAL

Looking out of the window over the expanse of the Labrador Sea, I can see snowmobiles below screaming across the ice in the bitter cold. Our ultimate destination lies more than fifty kilometres away, out on that frozen sea ice, where a dramatic battle between climate change and the Inuit people's way of life unfolds with each passing winter.

The plane skims along the frozen ocean, aiming for the narrow runway extending from the shoreline. We brace ourselves for the slippery landing on the icy gravel runway. The wheels touch down, and the engine revs to slow the aircraft, lurching us forward as a distant fence rapidly approaches. Inside the cabin, there's a feeling of palpable relief as the door opens for us to deplane. Exiting, we witness the typical roles of passengers, pilots, and baggage handlers blur into a collective effort. Everyone pitches in to unload the luggage, forming an impromptu team on the snow-covered tarmac. The ticket agent fuels the plane; the pilots toss us our bags while the next guests casually board, selecting their seats as if on a public bus.

Our hosts from the town, decked out in snowsuits and standing ready with their snowmobiles, greet us with a warm hug. As we load our gear onto the komatik—a sled drawn by a snowmobile—I feel a pang of embarrassment. Earlier, I'd asked about the possibility of a taxi or car rental, which I now see is ludicrous. With its small radius and snow-covered roads, Nain doesn't accommodate any vehicle other than the nimble snowmobiles that dart along the streets with a steady throttle of engines.

As we bump along the icy path, Braeden and James perch precariously atop the komatik with our luggage and exchange apprehensive glances. Each

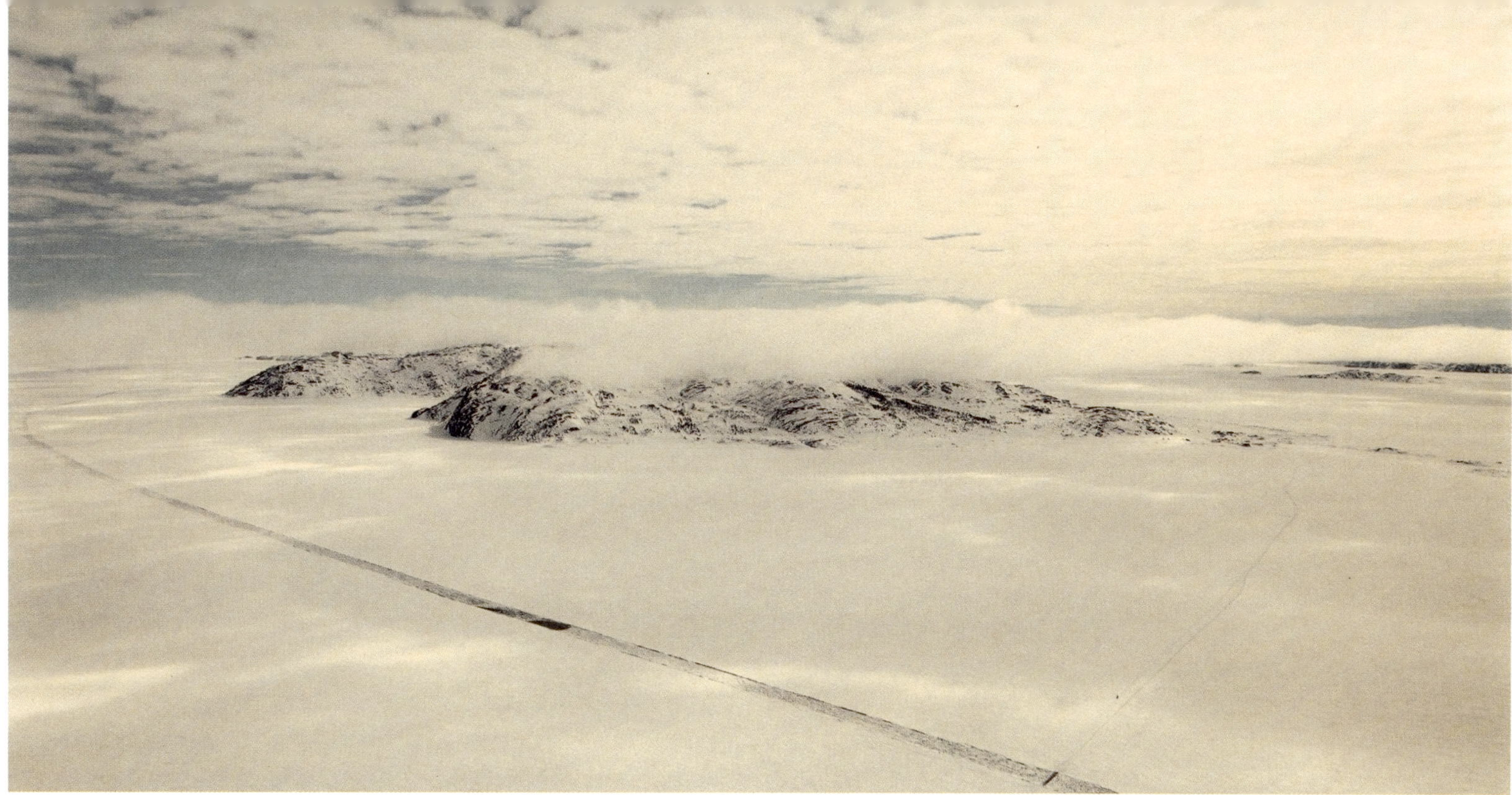

bounce causes a nervous laugh as they flip-flop between the novelty of the experience and concern over fragile camera gear. I watch their faces light up with the thrill of the unfamiliar as I hold on tight to our driver.

The hotel we check into is an experience in and of itself, a recently renovated structure standing in stark contrast to the town's simple surroundings. Its eerie emptiness, punctuated only by the manager's overly enthusiastic welcome, adds an element of suspense to our subarctic journey. Weather disruptions from the previous week had left many visitors stranded, we learn, and the prospect of an impending storm suggests that we, too, might be extending our stay, much to the apparent delight of our hosts.

We spend our first evening exploring Nain, starting with a visit to the Illusuak Cultural Centre to learn more about the traditional Inuit way of life and the long history of the land. Then we wander toward the shore, captivated by the snowmobiles streaking along the sea ice. Their constant flow resembles a highway that extends to the unknown expanse beyond the bay.

Our stroll leads us to the local grocery store, where the high prices are a sobering testament to the socio-economic challenges the people of the North face. We get a small bag of food, and the bill comes in at a staggering $140. The steep costs of transporting food to such remote regions lead to stark inequity for residents when compared to our lives back home. This, coupled with the additional pressure from climate change on their traditional ways of life, creates a specific and precarious vulnerability for the community.

As we trudge back to the hotel in the biting cold, the 4:00 p.m. sunset casts long, spectral shadows on the snow. A sense of unease seems to trail us back on the empty streets as stories of polar bears and wolves race in our minds. The echo of the ghostly, quiet hotel corridors compounds our anxiety as the repetition of rooms with no occupants seems endless. It feels otherworldly, like something out of a Stephen King novel. I fumble with my room key, overtaken by the urge to quickly escape the hallway's cold emptiness and retreat to the comfort of my room.

This is the far North, where beauty is woven with harsh reality, and resilience is a way of life. It is a place that humbles the unfamiliar, challenging preconceived notions and offering a powerful perspective on the relationship between humans and the natural world.

[page 128] Sea Ice extending
[opposite] The ice breaker trail 50 km out to sea; [above] Checking the Ice Buoy

INTO THE NORTH

The following day, we plan to leave the sheltered harbour of Nain and head out onto the sea ice. I want to witness firsthand the impact of a warming climate on northern and Arctic regions. Once a sturdy and reliable highway connecting remote communities, the sea ice is thinning in the face of warming ocean currents, and the people who rely on it face the daunting reality of losing not just a way to get around, but a way of life that is vital to their health and well-being.

Today, we are joining forces with Rex and his team at SmartIce. The initiative, a ground-breaking project hailed as the world's first climate change adaptation tool, combines traditional knowledge of ice with advanced data acquisition and remote monitoring technology. It provides near real-time insights into sea-ice thickness and local ice conditions. SmartIce involves a business model intent on preserving local cultures and lifestyles.

Rex's love for his community and land is palpable as he welcomes me into the facility. His cheerful personality balances the gravity of our expedition. Rex is not just a guide or a community leader; he is at the forefront of studying a warming world. As an Inuk—a member of the Labrador Inuit community—Rex is wholly committed to the work as a way of preserving his heritage.

As he graciously shows us around the location, a modest structure that combines a workshop and storage area, it becomes apparent why the community of Nain is so invested in the SmartIce project from a cultural perspective. The walls are covered with posters showcasing various processes, students' progress, and news clippings highlighting the company's accomplishments. As we admire the displays, Rex talks about the youth involved in the program and the pride he takes in mentoring the next generation. He emphasizes the vital importance of the program, which keeps those travelling on the sea ice safe and preserves tradition, particularly in the face of the changing climate.

"Each year, our harbour freezes over later than usual. We've even experienced rain as late as January, and the ice doesn't fully form until a month later than it used to," Rex explains earnestly. "Our seasons are shifting, and warmer summers have shortened our time on the ice. That's why we want you to be here, to share our story and raise awareness that climate change is real. While it may not affect everyone in the same noticeable way, it's impacting our community. Ice is more than just a highway for us—it's our way of life, it's our culture."

With that, Rex motions for us to get set up. We position an ice sensor that securely fastens to the komatik behind his snowmobile. Rex pulls out his iPad, checking the readings to ensure everything is in order. Recognizing—and slightly entertained by—our attempt to dress appropriately for the harsh northern climate, Rex hands us fleece face coverings branded with the SmartIce logo. "These will help keep you warm," he says with a smile. His face, weathered by the wind and marked with goggle lines from days when the snow made navigation challenging, speaks of his familiarity with the elements.

Joining us today is Richard, also a member of the Inuit community and part of the team at SmartIce. He is in his mid-thirties and emanates a sense of confidence around his role. He wears worn seal-skin mitts and a thick camouflage jacket. He doesn't wear goggles or a hat as the balmy negative ten degrees Celsius is far from the depth of winter cold he is used to. His snow-

[opposite] Sled from above

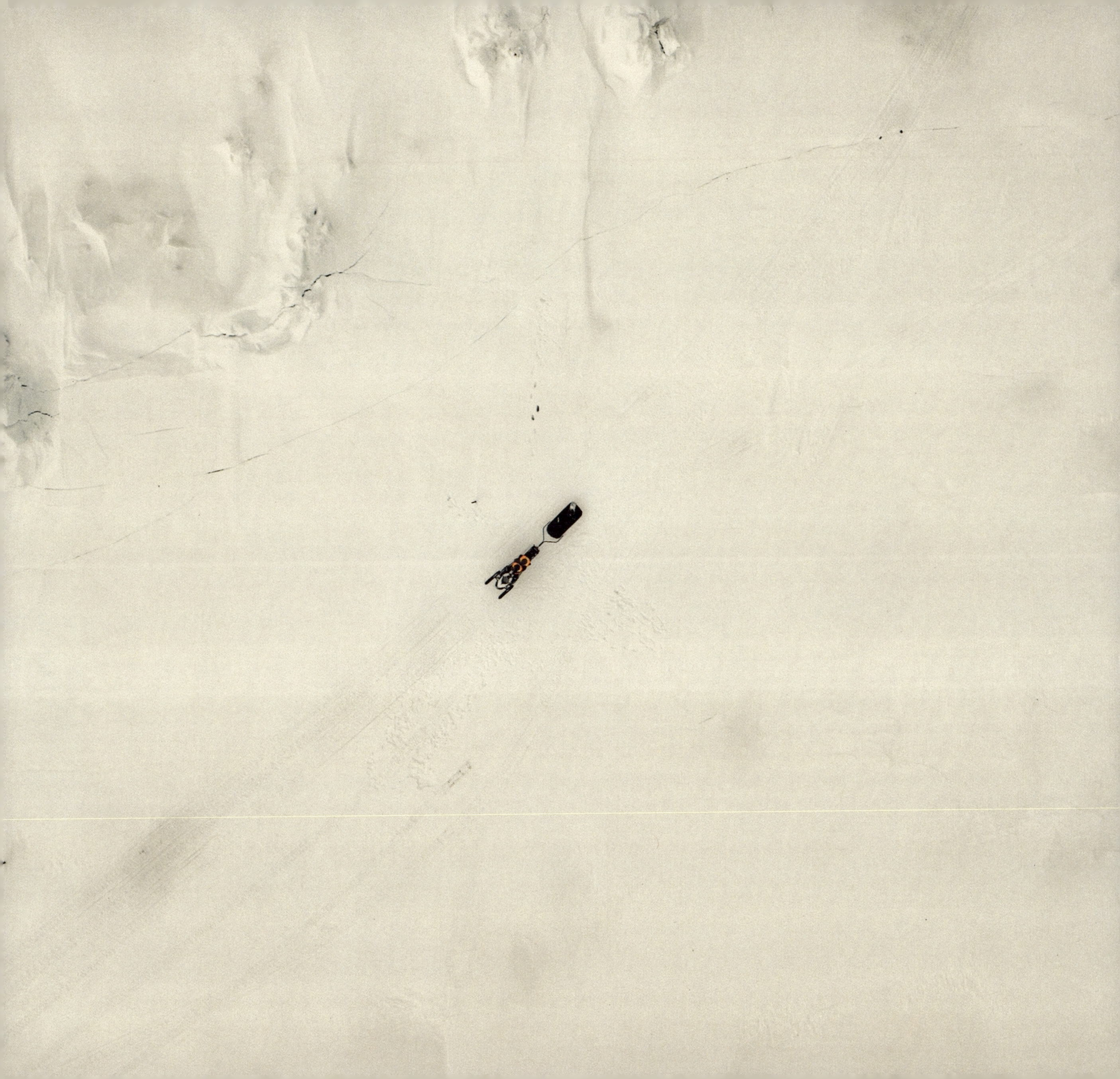

mobile is black and red and resembles a stealth bomber. It is perfectly maintained, clearly a prized possession. He smokes a cigarette as he shares tales of the Cain's Quest competition. Considered the most gruelling and dangerous snowmobile competition in the world, the race sees participants travel more than 3,000 kilometres across the whole of Labrador. Amazed, I bombard him with questions about how he could compete, which he shrugs off with humility, indicating that it was an expectation when coming from this area. He was raised in Nain and has travelled on the sea ice his entire life.

They start their snowmobiles, and I hop on behind Rex, ready to embark on our expedition.

Today, Rex and his team will show us how the thinning ice leads to increasingly unsafe travel conditions. What was once a reliable pathway has become treacherous and unpredictable, with hidden cracks and unstable surfaces that can result in accidents, injuries, or even fatalities.

As our snowmobiles race across the powdery surface, the wind howls with a bone-chilling intensity. The exposed skin on our faces goes numb. While our local guides see this as a warm spring day, for those of us venturing from distant cities, it is a bitterly cold adventure, a bracing taste of a world few of us have even imagined. Giant ice crystals erupt from below, like frozen sentinels, as if nature is defiantly resisting the encroaching warmth. Each icy shard magnifies the rocks beneath the frozen sea, a poignant reminder of the delicate balance between the sea ice and the hidden shore.

The landscape unfolds in an awe-inspiring panorama—an expansive archipelago of islands and bays adorned with rocky, barren cliffs blend with the frozen sea. This desolate beauty holds the wisdom of a timeless way of life. Yet, as we traverse the ice, an undeniable truth lingers in the air, mingling with the bitter cold. It whispers of impending tragedy, of an irreversible transformation of the ice and the path we travel.

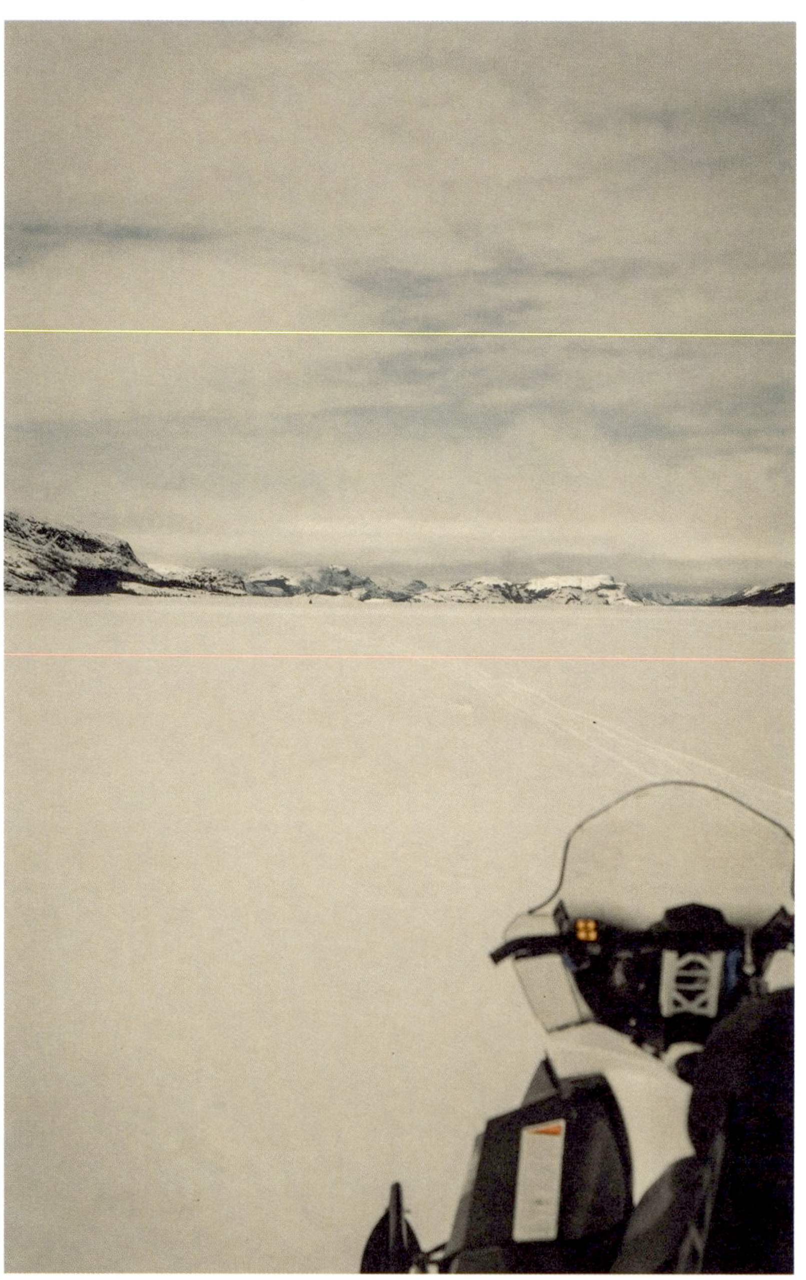

[above] The highway
[opposite] In the snow

Above us, the clouds race across the sky, casting somber shadows on the ice below. But even in that gloom, rays of sunlight pierce through, offering moments of warmth on our faces, reminding us of the intricate dance between a warming planet and these icy realms.

Guided by our local companions, we speed confidently across the ice, absorbing their tales and deep connection to this vast, untamed wilderness. "This is where we gather wood," Rex shares, pointing to a distant shore. "Over there is a hole in the ice where we hunt seals," he reveals, his voice filled with reverence for the ancient traditions intertwined with the ice. Yet, beneath the surface of excitement, an unease gnaws at my thoughts. These resilient people, the Inuit, bear the weight of climate change's side effects despite having played no part in its creation. To call it unfair is the grandest of understatements.

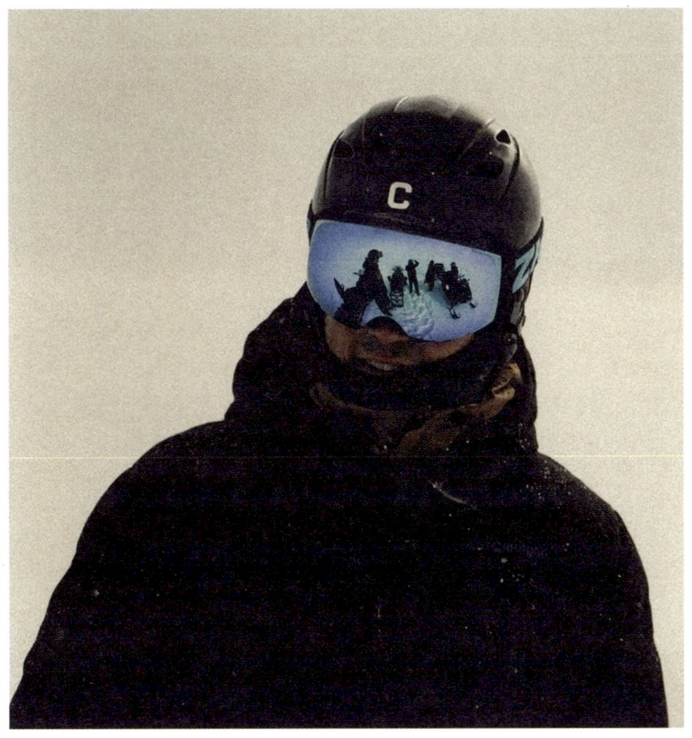

As we journey deeper into the ice-covered landscape, the implications of climate change on the health of the Inuit community become increasingly apparent. Sea ice has always been an integral part of their existence, providing a means for transportation, hunting, and fishing—crucial activities that feed them and nourish their cultural identity, and physical and mental well-being. The decline in sea ice disrupts these traditional activities, putting food security at risk by preventing the community from accessing traditional food sources like seals and fish.

The Inuit, so long sustained by the nutritional abundance of marine foods, find their health jeopardized as they are forced to shift toward imported, often processed, foods. This leads to a rise in chronic diseases such as obesity, diabetes, and heart disease.

The lack of safe ice also restricts access to remote cabins and recreational areas, leading to confinement and isolation in a community accustomed to free movement. The unforgiving mountains that encircle Nain, symbols of the region's natural beauty, start to feel like impassable barriers. This loss of mobility leads to heightened stress, anxiety, and other mental health issues.

But as the ice diminishes, so too do the bonds that tie the Inuit to their ancestral ways. The very essence of their cultural identity is under siege. For generations, the Inuit people have thrived in harmony with the ice, its presence woven into their traditions, practices, and collective memory.

Their health is inextricably tied to the health of the sea ice, and I realize that Rex, along with everyone in his community, is watching its disappearance take its toll. The loss of hunting grounds, the disappearance of familiar landscapes, and the erosion of vital skills chip away at their cultural fabric, leaving a void that echoes with sadness and frustration. This emotional burden must be borne by the community as the people grapple with the realization that the very spirit of who they are is slipping away.

A SOBERING REALITY

In that numbing cold my mind begins to wander, leaving behind the vast expanse of the sea ice as it drifts back to the warmer confines of the Canadian Museum of Nature in Ottawa, and I recall entering the grand museum with countless displays of Canada's natural heritage.

Dr. Jeff Saarela, an esteemed botanist and an expert on Arctic plant life, was my guide that day. Scholarly but seasoned in fieldwork, he struck me as a perfect combination of adventurer and researcher. Jeff seeks to understand the relationships between the changing temperatures and the Arctic through his work. By studying grasses, sedges, and their relatives from the Canadian Arctic, he can paint a picture of how this area is experiencing rapid environmental change.

When we arrived, Jeff took us to an exhibit named "Beyond Ice." This unique installation, a collaboration between the Canadian Museum of Nature and the National Film Board of Canada, features a series of large ice sculptures that echo the Arctic lands being swept away by disruptive forces. Visitors are encouraged to touch the ice to witness the transformation as it melts, revealing images and stories of the landscapes and living organisms inhabiting the northern regions. The day we planned to visit, ironically, the "Beyond Ice" display had literally melted—a metaphor too poignant to ignore.

Next, we ventured into the Arctic gallery, where interactive exhibits depicted a timeline of temperature changes over the Arctic's geological history. During my visit to that gallery, it became all too clear: The Arctic was warming at an unprecedented rate. Temperatures are rising and sea ice is declining. In 2020, the Arctic's minimum sea ice extent was the second lowest on record since satellite observations began in 1979. And the trend is strong: The fourteen lowest extents in the satellite record have occurred in the last fourteen years. The permafrost is also thawing. By the late 2010s, the Arctic was losing around 1.2 trillion metric tons of ice every year—equivalent to 300 million Olympic swimming pools. Worse, the top three metres of permafrost soil contains about 1,580 gigatons of carbon, which is almost twice the amount of carbon currently in the atmosphere. As the permafrost thaws, that carbon is released.

That museum visit, that crucial conversation with Dr. Saarela, became the catalyst for my journey to the North. I wanted to stand on the sea ice and see the changes for myself. I needed to understand the impact firsthand.

Fast forward to this present moment. I am thousands of kilometres north of the museum, standing on the very ice depicted in its exhibits.

Our destination comes into view, a solitary ice buoy station amid the endless frozen sea. As Rex sets up, he shares how the equipment works and points out that we have been moving along a frequently travelled ice highway, which is why the buoy is placed in its location. It is also close to a small bridge, which divides the ice with an open-water channel carved by the ships that travel to the mine down the coast.

As we stand on the ice, Rex directs our attention to the ice thickness sensor. It's a sobering moment. Their ice drills and measurements transform the abstract concept of a changing Arctic into a tangible, undeniable reality.

Then he demonstrates how he uploads the data to the server. This valuable information plays a critical role in ensuring the safety of travellers, alerting them to any potentially hazardous areas. Curious about the necessity of such technology in the past, I ask Rex for his insight.

"In the past, this type of technology wasn't available, but it certainly would have made a difference," Rex responds. He emphasizes the inherent dangers of the ice and the unpredictable nature of the landscape, highlighting the need for as much information as possible. "With the sea ice thinning, monitoring becomes even more important. The Inuit people possess ancestral knowledge of the ice and combining that knowledge with data allows them to make informed decisions about travel and hunting."

As his words resonate, I feel I am beginning to grasp the true significance of ice in Inuit culture. It becomes clear that this technology has the potential not only to help protect their cultural heritage but also to ensure their safety in this unforgiving environment. The integration of traditional wisdom and scientific data is a powerful combination, offering a path forward in navigating the changing Arctic landscape while preserving the invaluable knowledge passed down through generations.

As we continue our journey across the ice, the weight of responsibility stays with me. Each metre we travel creates a measurement we upload to the server. Our trip becomes more than a visit to the buoy; it is a small act of service to the community that has welcomed us so warmly. We are able to take part in a commitment to honouring the past while embracing the possibilities of the future.

This is a unique aspect of preserving health I didn't expect to experience. It is the intersection of tradition and technology forging a path of sustainability and strength in the face of an uncertain tomorrow.

On our way back, Rex lets me take the reins of the snowmobile as we cross the narrow bridge over the open water below, a reprieve from an endless expanse of frozen ocean. As I drive across a landscape so beautiful and foreign to me, I reflect on the experience of the day. I can't forget what I have learned and how I've been, briefly, not merely a spectator but a participant. With Rex's guidance, I have become a witness, opening my eyes and seeing a world on the brink of life-altering change for the first time. Understanding the situation, like the ice beneath our sleds, is necessary.

What if this delicate equilibrium shatters before we can fix it? What does it mean for the people of the North who rely on the ice for sustenance, transportation, and culture? And what does it mean for the world beyond the icy expanse? These questions, haunting and urgent, reverberate, inviting me to confront the far-reaching consequences of a changing climate on a global scale.

The story unfolding in the North serves as a stark warning as to the impact our decisions have on our world and its people.

Climate change is a health issue, and a dire one. The Inuit are already on the front lines and grappling with the growing impacts on their physical and mental health. The same challenges they face—dwindling sources of healthy food, a weakened ecosystem, and threatened cultural traditions—may look different farther south, but will expose everyone on the planet to the risks of climate change sooner or later.

The fate of our planet rests in our collective hands. We all share a responsibility to use this knowledge to foster a sustainable future that includes the survival of the sea ice, the Arctic, and, ultimately, our planet.

TAKE ACTION

REDUCE, REUSE, RECYCLE: Adopt an attitude that challenges our throw-away society and repurpose whenever possible. What is left should be recycled. Reused and recycled items create far fewer emissions (and reduce the use of virgin materials and the strain on landfills). Create an organized system to ensure you do your part.

CONSERVE WATER AND ELECTRICITY: Simple changes like turning off lights when leaving a room, unplugging electronics, taking shorter showers, capturing rainwater, and watering gardens with hoses designed to reduce water usage all achieve this goal. Remember, clean fresh water is a limited resource, and most energy is generated from non-renewable resources with high carbon footprints.

SUPPORT SUSTAINABLE FOOD SYSTEMS: Buy local when you can, join a community garden, or go to the farmers' market. This will not only support our local farmers, foragers, and food producers, but it will also reduce the carbon emissions associated with long-distance transport and non-sustainable farming practices.

EDUCATE YOURSELF ON CLIMATE CHANGE: Take time to learn about the environmental issues affecting your community. Have conversations and see what people are doing to help—you may find a whole new community (and some friends) equally committed to helping our environment.

SUPPORT INDIGENOUS-LED INITIATIVES: Support Indigenous businesses, organizations, and community groups making a difference. Indigenous cultures have a unique and well-developed perspective on the land, water, and air, and can offer sustainable alternatives to current practices.

OUR CLIMATE CHAMPIONS

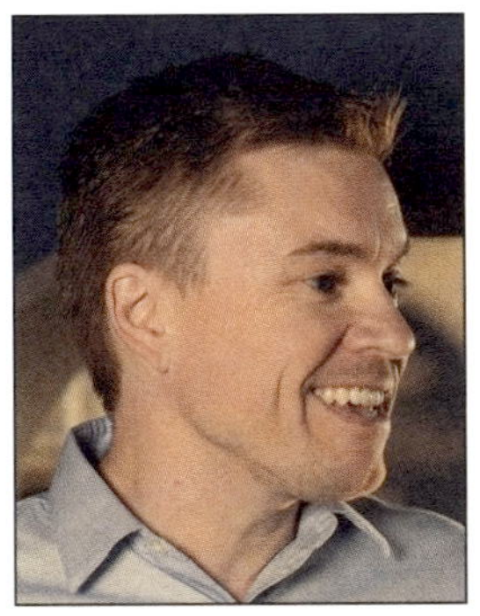

DR. JEFF SAARELA: Serving as the director of Research at the Canadian Museum of Nature, Dr. Saarela has committed his professional life to investigating the implications of climate change on the varied plant life indigenous to the Arctic. He underscores that while the progression of climate change might seem gradual and almost imperceptible to many of us, year after year, it is manifesting at a pace accelerated more than any other period in our history.

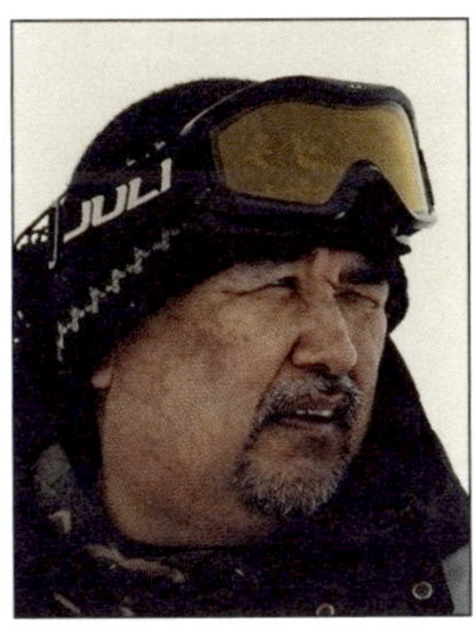

REX HOLWELL: A deeply rooted member of the Inuit community, Rex sincerely understands the ice and its role in the Inuit way of life. His passion for training youth and preserving their traditions is his motivation for the SmartIce project. We are grateful to Rex for sharing with us so much about this community and the pressures the Inuit face, and guiding us across the vast expanse of the frozen Labrador Sea.

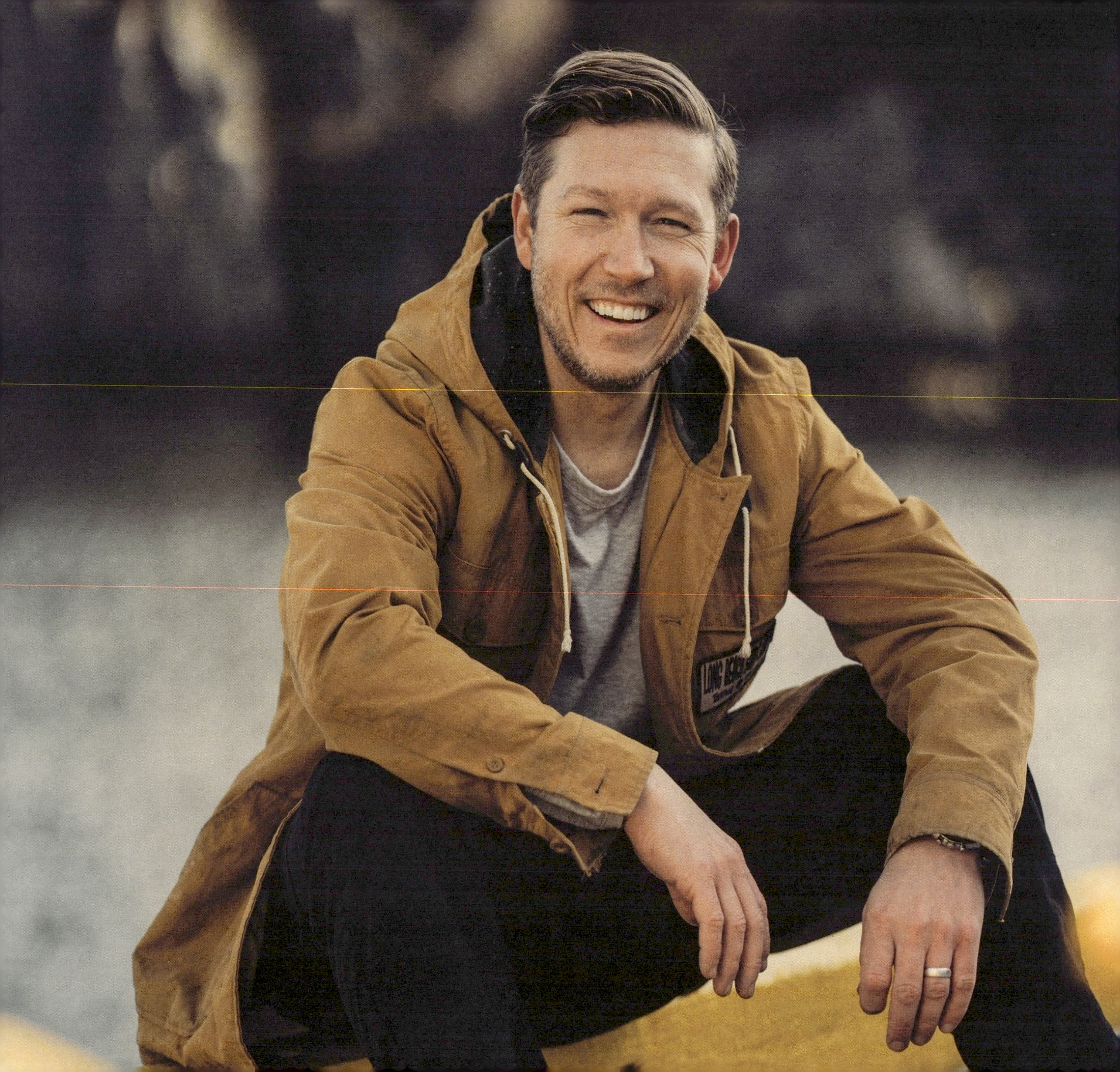

COMING HOME

My journey around the globe has been a quest for understanding health in its truest sense. I've realized that health is much more than a physical state—it's rooted in our peace of mind, our happiness, and the strength of our communities. Our health is shaped by who we are, where we dwell, our beliefs, and the values we cherish. It's fostered by the environment we create around ourselves and the people we choose to share our lives with.

Throughout my career, I have sought to empower others with knowledge, simplifying the complex health landscape to help people make informed, individualized decisions. My travels, enriched by diverse global perspectives, reinforced my belief that health is a personal journey of balance and understanding.

This journey has led to some amazing adventures and given me an incredible sense of achievement. But my greatest achievement is waiting for me at home. It is one that came later in life when the headstrong nature of youth matured and life calmed. It was meeting my wife, who changed everything for me. Despite almost twenty years of familiar friends, shared interests, and social events, we had never met. Now I realize this delay in our encounter was all a part of the plan, a chance to meet when the timing was right. And when the time came, our connection was instantaneous and magical.

I'm flying home now, and the empty seat beside me makes my anticipation to see her grow. I'm returning to what truly matters—the love of my life and the close-knit community that is my anchor.

As I look out of the plane window, it's not just the world below that captivates me; it's what I have learned along the way. This journey home is not just a physical return but an arrival to a new understanding of what health means to me.

The rocky cliffs of my home appear through the clouds, and I know I'm done with merely gazing out of windows, always searching for something more. My travels have taught me to embrace a peaceful and contented life. I am returning to the place I call home, ready to enjoy a sustainable, healthy, and happy life surrounded by love and a sense of belonging.

[opposite] Mike Wahl, home in Newfoundland

acknowledgements

I remember digging through a box of abandoned books I had discovered in the attic of my first rented apartment. I was far from home, working my first job just outside of New York City. I was unaccustomed to being alone, and in my uneasy boredom, an attic ladder called me to explore what was above. A book with a red cover caught my eye, open and inviting me to read, left by some unknown messenger. That was my introduction to *A Psalm of Life* by Henry Wadsworth Longfellow—each line of the prose awoke the motivation that lay dormant inside me. It is an inspiring tale of what life could and should be, one that is inquisitive, searching, and patient; words that I needed at that moment. I still have that book at home and reflect on it often.

I have been lucky to share my life journey with countless unique souls. Some have been constant characters in my story, while others have passed through with glimmers of wisdom that have altered my course ever so slightly. They have provided a nudge that sets me on the right track, where travel is smoother, a slipstream of fulfillment.

I find life fascinating, not only the experience but also its function. It's captivating how our bodies can operate without any guidance from us, how they grow and heal, age and change. This curiosity about the inner and outer world has led me to this point.

I have had guides along my journey who have left footsteps for me to follow, mentors like my mother, Sharon, and father, John, who have always encouraged me to pursue my dreams, constantly stoking my enthusiasm and masterfully pushing me to succeed in the most supporting ways. My wife and soulmate, Leanne, who has inspired me to pen my thoughts and share my story. Your belief in me and your companionship has given me the courage to create a life that is lived to the fullest. Seeing the world through the lens of your love has changed my perspective and helped me see the beauty around me.

To my closest friends who consistently inspire me with their craft: Don E. Coady, communicator extraordinaire; Stephen Henley, a voice of logic and stoicism; Dr. Hasan Khalili, adventurer and sage; Kevin Peters, shed philosopher; Rich Haywood, whose competition for the best stories fuels me to experience more; and lastly, we are grateful to Brian Henley for believing in us and this project—thank you all for being exactly who you are.

I have to recognize my scholarly mentors: Dr. David Behm, who has become family to me and shown me what a true education in life means, and Dr. Gerry Mugford, who saw unorthodox as valuable and encouraged me to stay the course of my doctorate when I was travelling on the darkest of roads. You inspire me to teach like you do and impact those around me.

There is a saying that there is no sweet without sour, no wave without a trough, and no mountain without a valley. I am grateful for those who have taught me the hardest lessons and allowed me to appreciate the full spectrum of the human experience.

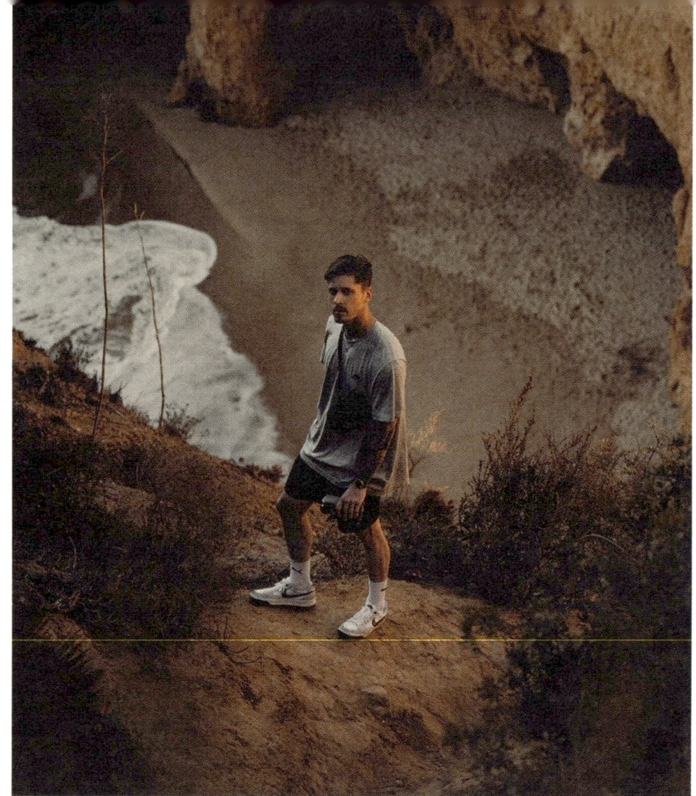

[above] Braeden King
[opposite] Entrance to Meiji Jingu gardens

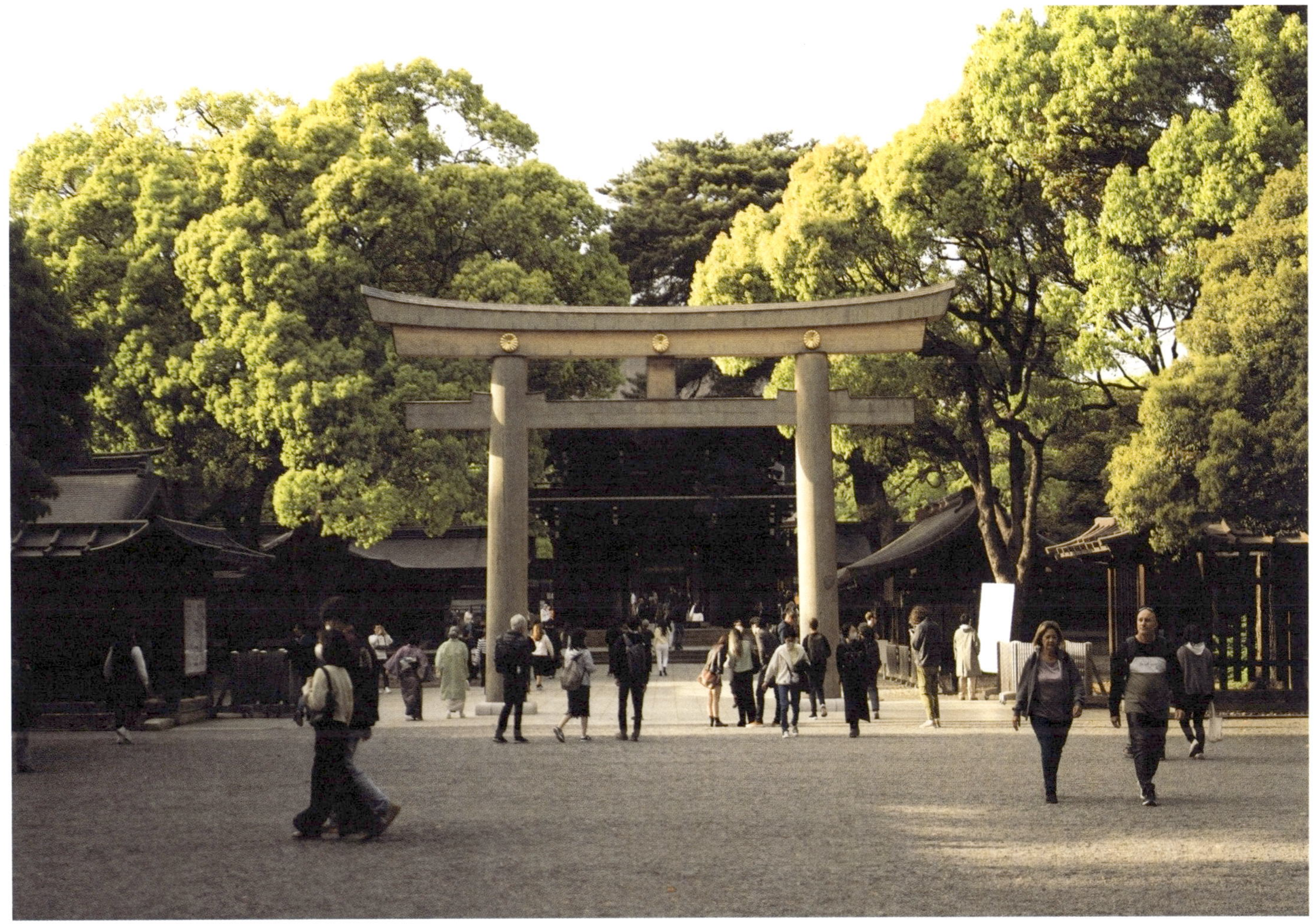

To my students and academic colleagues, who motivate me with curiosity and impress me with their knowledge, I am grateful to have you as a reminder of why we do what we do. Thank you to Memorial University for letting me focus my efforts on projects that educate our community and share the human story. Likewise, to those in the arts who provided me the platform to follow my dreams to create—Jesse Stirling and family, Jonathan Mercer, Fabian James, James MacKinnon, and Jacob Critch—thank you for believing in this mission.

To my editor, Leslie Vryenhoek, who has kindly provided feedback and coached me on how to write, and Rebecca Rose and the team at Breakwater for adopting this work. Your confidence in me has fuelled my writing.

To the elders, teachers, guides, and all the incredible people I have met around the world, thank you for inviting me into your homes, sharing your life's work, and trusting me with your secrets of life; I only hope I have done your teachings justice. Those moments spent in conversation are treasures I will value my entire life.

Lastly, I want to thank Braeden for his creativity, growth, and commitment as we traversed the globe and become better humans for it. We have captured the moments in our own ways and now can share those perspectives with others in the hopes that they may, too, take the leap and do something daring.

biographies

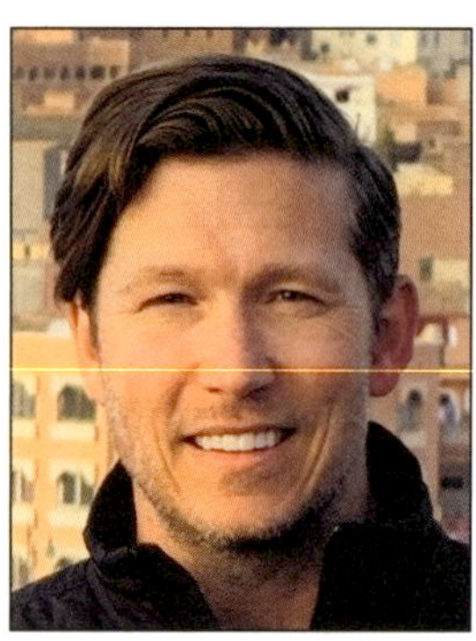

DR. MIKE WAHL, a professor of medicine at Memorial University, has always had a passion for health education. His twenty-five-year career spans academia, media, and entrepreneurship on a global scale. He is an explorer, having traversed over fifty countries, a speaker, and a documentary filmmaker for the series *Health Explored*, which shares unique insights into health practices worldwide. His work emphasizes a commitment to advancing health and wellness understanding, and inspiring individuals to contemplate what health means to them.

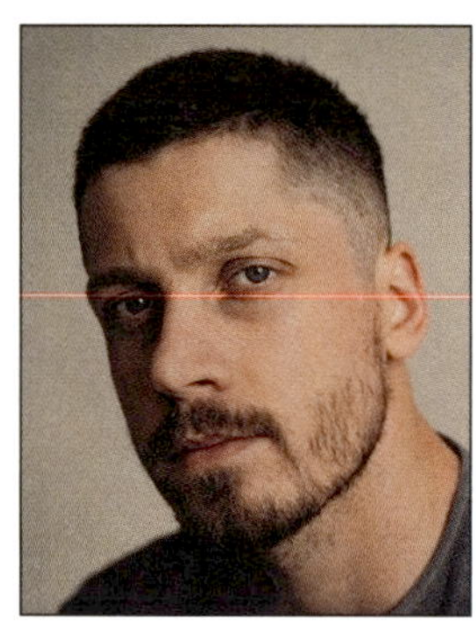

BRAEDEN KING is a self-taught photographer, director, and world traveller. His passion for visual arts has led him to collaborate with individuals and organizations worldwide. His work has been featured by *Canadian Geographic*, *Discovery Channel*, the United Nations, *Lonely Planet*, and Parks Canada. He finds joy in capturing unique stories of inspiring individuals and sharing rare moments from parts of the globe only seen by few. Braeden is a professional in the art of creativity.